Girls and Their Monsters

Also by Audrey Clare Farley

The Unfit Heiress: The Tragic Life and Scandalous Sterilization of Ann Cooper Hewitt

Girls and Their Monsters

The Genain Quadruplets and the Making of Madness in America

Audrey Clare Farley

GRAND CENTRAL

New York Boston

Grand Central Publishing
Hachette Book Group
1290 Avenue of the Americas, New York, NY 10104
grandcentralpublishing.com
twitter.com/grandcentralpub

First Edition: June 2023

Grand Central Publishing is a division of Hachette Book Group, Inc. The Grand Central Publishing name and logo is a trademark of Hachette Book Group, Inc.

The publisher is not responsible for websites (or their content) that are not owned by the publisher.

The Hachette Speakers Bureau provides a wide range of authors for speaking events. To find out more, go to hachettespeakersbureau.com or email HachetteSpeakers@hbgusa.com.

Grand Central Publishing books may be purchased in bulk for business, educational, or promotional use. For information, please contact your local bookseller or the Hachette Book Group Special Markets Department at special.markets@hbgusa.com.

Print book interior design by Marie Mundaca

Library of Congress Cataloging-in-Publication Data
Names: Farley, Audrey Clare, author.
Title: Girls and their monsters: the Genain quadruplets and the making of madness in America / Audrey Clare Farley.
Description: New York, NY: Grand Central Publishing, [2023]
Identifiers: LCCN 2022057896 | ISBN 9781538724477 (hardcover) | ISBN 9781538724491 (ebook)
Subjects: LCSH: Quadruplets—United States. | Schizophrenia—United States. | Mental health—United States.
Classification: LCC HQ777.35 .F37 2023 | DDC 306.8750973—dc23/eng/20230111
LC record available at https://lccn.loc.gov/2022057896
ISBNs: 978-1-5387-2447-7 (hardcover), 978-1-5387-2449-1 (ebook)

Printed in the United States of America

LSC-C

Printing 1, 2023

For Sarah

Girls and Their Monsters

History always comes home to roost. There is no possibility of a life uncompromised by the violence of the past.

Olivia Laing, *Everybody: A Book About Freedom*

Prologue

Edna is the first to come downstairs. Being the eldest, she's the spokesperson for the group. She's somewhat haggard looking, the psychiatrist in the living room notes. "Might be more attractive under more favorable circumstances," he writes.

Next is Wilma. She used to be the clown of the family, but these days she's in a catatonic stupor. Her mother explains that she will find a place in the house and then root herself there, unfazed by the surrounding commotion. She tires from standing so many hours, even at night. When she sinks into a tattered chair now, it is for the first time all day.

Helen is right behind Wilma. She's unkempt in a Cinderella-by-the-fire manner. Her garments don't fit, and there's a hole at one elbow. Her pupils are enlarged, and she keeps fiddling with imaginary objects before her mother can grab her hands and return them to her sides.

Finally there's Sarah. She's well groomed, though the circles of rouge against her white cheeks give her a china-doll quality. The "sweetest of the four," but a bit "mechanical and hollow," the psychiatrist thinks. Everything about her seems "real, but not quite."

When all of the twenty-four-year-old quadruplets have taken their seats, the visitor finds his attention drawn to Helen, who resembles a twisted coil. She bends to conform to her chair, then spontaneously springs in different directions. As the parents, Carl and Sadie Morlok, begin to make small talk, the psychiatrist's eyes drift toward the pictures hanging on the wall. All of the sisters in childhood. In the adjoining dining room, he can see the couch-bed and the hook with trousers and ties, and he wonders if Carl sleeps downstairs. Then, as if on cue, Sadie reaches for a photograph album and begins to reminisce about the days when the quadruplets toured the country as a singing and dancing troupe. She and her daughters applaud at certain pictures and bend over others, momentarily confused about who's who. It seems like they're all used to the routine, like they've done this skit before.

Mrs. Morlok boasts that she was the quadruplets' stage manager, and the psychiatrist considers how masterfully she must have executed that role. In his view, she's "like the center of a five-spoked wheel, turning the family in one direction or another." She also has something of a "property-possession attitude to the girls." When she briefly leaves the room to take Helen to the bathroom, Sarah assumes the role of hostess. There seems to be a sense of surrogacy in her performance. But when Carl speaks from the other side of the room, she immediately grows quiet, nodding at whatever he has to say. She does not dare to interrupt him except to supply a name on the tip of his tongue. He, too, seems to regard his daughters as objects.

The patriarch has a bulbous nose and an anxious manner that the visitor will remember. Before he called the sisters downstairs, Carl had referred to his "condition" several times. He meant his diabetes. Perhaps he wanted his visitor to know the quadruplets weren't the only ones with ailments. He was affable enough, if not as welcoming as his wife, who spoke plainly of being rescued by the doctor and his colleagues. Mrs. Morlok explained that she was convalescing from a bladder operation and could not continue to run a psychiatric ward. Her husband seemed defeated that it had come to this.

The conversation moves to the prospect of the sisters traveling east to be studied. It's evident the parents have already broached the subject with the quadruplets. Mrs. Morlok mentions sightseeing and dancing, perhaps even the occasion for a professional comeback for the troupe. Edna, the eldest, is visibly unconvinced. According to Mrs. Morlok, she's terribly attached to their psychiatrist. As she's being talked about, Edna begins to grimace and flex her hands. Out of politeness, the visitor turns to Wilma, asking how *she* feels about the proposed journey. "I can't answer him," she snaps, refusing to meet his eye.

Soon it's time for the young women's afternoon ritual: eggnog, barbiturates, and naps. Mr. Morlok has to hold the straw to Helen's lips, as she can no longer eat or drink on her own. This sister now appears to be actively hallucinating. When the Morloks begin to discuss Edna's eating habits, she nervously pushes her glass along the table, as if to distract from the subject. Complimented on her good behavior, Wilma stands and walks to the dining room, then fixes her limbs into a statue-like pose. Sarah, the china doll, continues to do and say the right things, but seems less and less alert as the minutes tick by. When the psychiatrist finally moves to leave, Mr. and Mrs. Morlok jump up to draw the chintz drapes. Clearly they are ready for the dreaming hour to begin.

Only two days later, the psychiatrist returns. This time the family is in beauty-parlor mode. Mrs. Morlok is putting Edna's hair in curlers, and Sarah is doing the same for Wilma, as Helen waits her turn. The two hairdressers next intend to bathe Edna and Helen, who are the least able to look after themselves. When it's mentioned that Edna and Helen were fighting the night before—Edna biting her nails down to the quick—Mr. Morlok tries to downplay their behaviors. He says many prominent people, including doctors, suffer from mental illness. If before he seemed resigned to his daughters being scrutinized by strangers, he now seems rather sore about the idea.

It's only after he has left for an appointment that his wife opens up. Mrs. Morlok describes him as a cantankerous person and confides that he's been trying to dissuade his eldest daughter from leaving home. Knowing Edna doesn't want to go, Carl goes on and on about how miserable she'll be. When Carl returns to the house, the psychiatrist gets him alone to hear his side of the story. The man only shrugs, as if the decision has already been made. Not long after this, the visitor takes his leave a second time, and both mother and father thank him for making arrangements for their daughters.

The visitor is Dr. Seymour Perlin from the National Institute of Mental Health (NIMH) in Bethesda, Maryland. He's traveled to Lansing, Michigan, to see the four sisters who've all been diagnosed with schizophrenia. Some of his colleagues back at NIMH are keen to demonstrate the genetic basis of the schizophrenia—something that would liberate the mind sciences from the grip of the childhood-obsessed neo-Freudians. Other colleagues remain interested in familial and internal conflicts. When the first group learned about the sisters from a Johns Hopkins University research psychologist named David Rosenthal, who is soon to join their ranks, they could hardly believe their good fortune. As far as they can tell, the estimated frequency of quadruplet births with at least one baby surviving is about one in a million. Only one in ten of those birth sets is monozygotic, meaning derived from the same ovum (and thus identical). While the proportion of quadruplet births with all four surviving is not documented, it is estimated to be about half, making the Morlok sisters one in approximately twenty million births. The chance of their *all* having schizophrenia is about one in one and a half billion. It's hard to imagine they will ever again have such an opportunity for study.

But these experts, who, along with their more environmentally attuned peers, will go on to contribute to Rosenthal's six-hundred-page book with the pseudonym title *The Genain Quadruplets: A Case Study and Theoretical Analysis of Heredity and Environment in Schizophrenia* (1963), are about to find that the matter of the sisters' madness is hardly so simple. Hours of doll play, Rorschach tests, handwriting analysis, psychotherapy sessions, and more will reveal the little clapboard two-story to be a house of horrors, making it difficult for researchers to draw any certain conclusions about either the origins or the nature of their shared disorder. Despite this, the book will propel the scientific community in one specific direction, and Rosenthal's life and career will never be the same.

For all their contributions to scientific literature, the NIMH researchers will leave some parts of the story untold. If the quadruplets' home was a mire of threats, so was the wider society in which they lived. Their great tragedy was having nowhere to rest. The danger was all around.

Perhaps the ubiquity of the violence the sisters endured is beyond these experts' pay grade. The hard scientists among them are trained to see human distress as something that arises from defective bodies, while the social scientists look no further than parental relationships, real or imagined. It may be that it's easier for the psyche, not just the scientific mind, to contend with disordered organs or families than with a disordered society. But the story of the Morlok sisters is the story of darkness coursing through the world. It's the story of malevolence masquerading as innocence and thereby hiding in plain sight. It's the story of a society professing great concern for its children, while actually exploiting them, and of the American family and other institutions compelling members to accept this and other societal contradictions, no matter the political or psychological costs.

Were experts to say that the quadruplets' whole milieu was perverse, they would have to consider that their tics bore witness to a pervasive truth, perhaps even that their tied tongues and deliria revealed more about the world than any written words. And that madness might come to take root in a person via society, which might then raise alarm about how porous *every* person was. After all, to let go of the unitary self—the notion that one is all alone in one's body—is both existentially frightening and ethically binding. Which would help to explain why investigators all over the world have long been feverish to define schizophrenia—to nail it down—despite how people always go crazy in their own way.

Most of the NIMH researchers will move on to other subjects, *The Genain Quadruplets* taking up just one line on the CV. A few will keep tabs on the sisters, either in the hope of discovering something even more scientifically momentous about them or, in Rosenthal's case, out of genuine concern. But not even this lead researcher will come to know everything about the foursome before tragedy strikes. Still their secrets will survive, on flesh and in hearts. They will haunt some, though they are everyone's to carry.

Chapter One

Sadie Lyon was only two years old when she learned to mother. At her family's rural Ohio farmhouse, she was put to work rocking the first of what would become six younger siblings. By four, she was changing diapers. By seven, cooking meals and milking cows. At that point, the babies were coming every two years.

Sadie could always tell *when* another one was coming—her mother would grow very sick and then swell in the abdomen—but she didn't know *where* they came from. Sometimes, when she noticed that both of her parents were absent, she would drift toward their bedroom to see what it was they were doing. Through the closed door she could hear them kissing. At nine, she once barged in to ask for help with the milking. She took one look at them tangled together, then ran to her own room. Soon after, her mother explained that babies came from eggs. Both a man and woman made an egg, and then the two eggs came together. When Sadie asked how they came together, her mother refused to answer. It wasn't until she began menstruating at eleven that her mother offered a few more details. After this, the birds and the bees were never spoken about again.

Decades later, some experts would wonder if it was such squeamishness about sex that blighted Sadie, if seeing and knowing—but having to pretend *not* to have seen and *not* to know—made her such a neurotic person. Freud described this dynamic in numerous patients who had stumbled across the "primal scene" as children.

Experts would also raise their eyebrows at Sadie's mother for enlisting her in the emotional labor of marriage. Mr. Lyon was extraordinarily moody. His wife always had to dote upon him to get him out of a funk. Afraid he might lash out at someone, Sadie helped her by paying him compliments or offering to fix his favorite drink. None of this ever endeared her to him. He scolded and degraded her, much preferring his sons and encouraging them in school. It was fine if his daughters didn't succeed, as they were only going to become homemakers. As far as he was concerned, they needed no more than an eighth-grade education.

Who could blame Sadie for seizing the chance to live with her maternal grandmother when both of her parents became ill, her father with sciatica and her mother with malaria? She dashed off to the home of Mrs. Amanda Meek in a village about eight miles away. Even after they both recovered, Sadie was allowed to stay with her grandmother as long as she returned home to help with the younger children on weekends and over the summers.

Her father always picked up where he left off. One day she decided she'd had enough of his insults. The now-fourteen-year-old packed her suitcase and went to tell her mother she was going back to her grandmother's for good. Her mother tried to dissuade her, but, seeing that Sadie had made up her mind, told her to make the most of things. That night her father appeared on his mother-in-law's doorstep with a shotgun in hand. Mrs. Meek refused to let him in. "I'll never help you with anything so long as you live," he shouted to Sadie through the screen door. "And you'll never again be welcome in the house." When she tried visiting her younger siblings a few years later, he reminded her of this promise.

Mrs. Meek permitted her to go out at night, though never alone with boys. Sadie and her peers wandered the fields laughing and carrying on. If she hadn't had bigger designs, she might have made a nice life there. But high school called, and she moved to another town with one to attend. At first, she worked as a telephone operator and waitress to pay for room and board in the new place. Then she became an assistant to a doctor. When the man's wife fell seriously ill, Sadie donated four pints of blood to save her life. In gratitude, he offered to pay for nursing school.

Nursing attracted Sadie, as it promised good wages *and* romance. Film and radio dramatized white-capped angels receiving wounded soldiers, then falling in love. Unfortunately she was never able to obtain her degree, as she couldn't pass Latin and chemistry. This was fine with her once she laid eyes on her employer's nephew, who was himself studying to be a doctor. Dr. Davenport, as he was called even then, was charming and kind. They would take vacations, posing as man and wife, and he eventually gave her a ring. Then one day he revealed that he had a heart condition. For her sake, he believed, they shouldn't marry. Her own heart broken, Sadie moved to the neighboring state of Michigan to work for a hospital physician as an unlicensed nurse. There she met the man who would put her on the map.

Carl Morlok had gone into the hospital for an appendectomy. Though he was loud and disgruntled, the other nurses were smitten. They liked the way he swore in German. Sadie didn't dare go near him, as she'd read a horoscope indicating that she'd wed a man with some of his negative characteristics. A few months later, she saw him at a baseball game and could feel him watching her.

She ran into him yet again at a house call. She and her employer, a doctor named LaBarge, were treating his brother Bill and his sister-in-law Loretta at their home for a venereal disease when Carl visited. Once he left, Loretta couldn't stop praising him. *Perhaps he's not so bad*, thought Sadie.

She'd do this over the years—let others write things in her head for the man instead of trusting her intuition. But in this case, her negative feelings resurged as Carl began to trail her like a puppy. She tried putting him off with a few curt remarks. When that didn't work, she became crueler. Even that didn't appear to bother him. The strange thing was that Sadie suspected him of returning his sister-in-law's affection. As she continued to treat Bill and Loretta, she sometimes caught him sitting on Loretta's bed, rubbing her back. Then Bill would enter the room, and he'd race out.

Sadie eventually agreed to go out with Carl, who was more than ten years her senior. He'd simply worn her down. She asked if there was anything between him and his sister-in-law, and he dodged the question. It was Loretta who confirmed her suspicions. "We've been having an affair," she bragged, "and if anything ever happens to Bill, we're going to be married."

Sadie decided it was best to be rid of Carl for good. If what Loretta said was true, he was probably diseased. But when she tried to end their courtship, he proposed marriage and threatened suicide if she refused. He also threatened to kill *her* if she ever spoke to his sister-in-law again. Loretta, for her part, cried at the news of the proposal. She'd never forgive Sadie for coming between her and Carl.

Years later, Sadie would regret that she didn't get out of town right then, instead soliciting the opinion of Dr. LaBarge. "He's of good people, if a little strange," said the physician.

"He's a drunkard," she replied. "He has only an eleventh-grade education. He's very domineering, and he'd be ugly to me if we married."

"You're too hard on him," said Dr. LaBarge.

Wanting some semblance of control, it seems, Sadie told Carl to stop drinking. He obeyed, and things improved between them. She agreed to obtain a marriage license, arranging for him to see LaBarge for a physical exam and blood test. If he tested positive for a venereal disease, she would have an excuse to back out, as it was frowned upon to pursue a union that wasn't "eugenically sound." But by some strange fortune, Carl checked out all right, and she went to buy a dress. His brother assured her she was doing the right thing.

If, after this, a final shudder passed through Sadie, she kept it to herself. They exchanged vows before a parson in a nearby town and then drove to her family's house, where a room had been prepared. Now that she was fulfilling her life's purpose, her father was willing to forget his grudge.

That night Carl paced the room with a nervous energy she'd never seen before. She'd later describe him as resembling a rabid dog. When the time came for intercourse, he wasn't the least bit gentle or affectionate. Just before he climaxed, he bit her face. Startled, she sat up in bed and clutched her bloody cheek as Carl settled into his pillow. Seeing him drift out of consciousness, she shook him and demanded to know what sort of spell he was having. In her own words, later offered to a social worker at NIMH, "he moaned and gave another snap of his teeth."

The next morning, when her mother called them down for breakfast, she hid under the blankets. She'd never felt so ashamed. She waited until her family left for a picnic to go downstairs.

"I'm sorry," said Carl. "I don't know why I did that."

They drove to see a physician, who patched her up and asked questions of the new groom. Sadie suspected epilepsy, but the doctor wasn't so sure. Then they made their way to the picnic, where she made excuses for her bandages. "A bad allergy," she told onlookers, the first of many lies for Carl.

That night her parents probed for the truth. She wanted to divulge what had actually happened, but couldn't bring herself to talk about something so impolite. Carl did not appreciate the tension. He soon claimed to be sick and demanded they leave for his mother's place back in Michigan.

Carl's mother, Katherine, left little question, at least in Sadie's mind, as to where he'd gotten his nastiness. The woman constantly criticized Sadie while praising her son "Collie." After putting Carl to work on home repairs, she would roam around asking, "What will I do without my Collie?" She also believed her own family to be racially superior. When Carl was three, the Morloks had emigrated from Germany and refused to mix with people who weren't German or even to speak English in the home. Katherine had told her children that people from other nationalities were responsible for America's troubles and so they should plan to marry someone with their own heritage. She had no problem expressing her disapproval of Sadie, whose ancestors were Scottish and Irish.

It was therefore a good thing for Sadie that they settled elsewhere. In the populous capital city of Lansing, home to several Oldsmobile plants, they rented an upstairs apartment and looked for work. Carl had wanted to stay in the countryside so he could fish and hunt rabbits, but there were more opportunities for her in the city. Sadie found work as a private nurse and then at St. Lawrence Hospital, where she quickly settled in. Carl, on the other hand, struggled to finish his shifts at his factory job. Every time someone looked at him the wrong way, he stormed out. As it was near the height of the Depression, there were always plenty of others to take his place.

The problems in the bedroom persisted. Sadie found that, like a werewolf who appeared on a full moon, Carl's "seizures" occurred between the seventeenth and twentieth days of the month. Once she deduced this, she made a habit of holding up a pillow to protect her face. Mostly she was uninterested in sex, but occasionally she would feel playful and try to initiate. Her overtures invariably repelled her husband, who once gasped in horror, "Are you in heat?"

Carl was absolutely opposed to having children, and Sadie agreed it was not a good idea. She and her husband barely spoke some nights, as she was always afraid of angering him. They didn't go out much, either, due to his jealousy over strangers talking to her. He'd accuse her of somehow knowing them behind his back. Wanting to experience a little joy in life, she signed up for a sewing class. Whenever she returned home from it, she'd find Carl standing in the window watching for her.

It wasn't his possessiveness that stirred Sadie to end things, but rather the occasional explosions between them. Once Carl's purchase of a new automobile set her off. He presented it to her for her birthday, but they both knew it was really for him. She demanded to know how he was going to pay for it. Carl admitted he was counting on her to take care of it. Sadie did have some savings from her employment with Dr. LaBarge, which he had actually hoped to live off before she'd coaxed him to find a job.

Sadie raced to the bedroom and proceeded to pack a suitcase for Carl. He accused her of being in a temper, and she backed down. Divorce was not really an attractive option. While Michigan law permitted it if one party was prone to drunkenness, congregants at the Emanuel First Lutheran Church she now attended might not be so understanding. The church was part of a very orthodox synod of evangelical Lutheranism, many of whose leaders viewed unsubordinated women as one of the world's greatest evils.

Another gift from her husband proved more favorable to the marriage. On their third anniversary in August 1929, he forgot to bring flowers or even acknowledge the occasion. "Well, you can give me a baby," she blurted. Sadie would later offer several reasons for her change of heart. In one version, she'd been told she was becoming menopausal and regretted not having children. In another, a doctor had advised that her uterus was out of position and only pregnancy could set it right. In yet another, she desired a baby because her husband withheld love. Whatever her motivations, she got her wish. That night, she and Carl had intercourse without using a contraceptive. The very next day, she knew it had worked: She had a magical feeling about her.

When her period didn't come a few days later, she went to see a Dr. Howard Haynes, who told her to come back in three weeks if she still hadn't bled. She waited the allotted time, during which Carl drank himself stupid, and then Dr. Haynes confirmed she was with child.

Not long after chills came and her skin turned purplish, she became convinced there were multiples. Dr. Haynes was not persuaded. "Aren't you a white woman?" he asked, parroting clinical and popular literature. Both portrayed people of color as hyper-breeders, often for the purposes of promoting forced sterilization laws.

At nine weeks, Sadie became unable to lie prostrate without choking. She couldn't urinate, and her kidneys were infected. All of her extremities were swollen, and she had a lot of vaginal discharge. Dr. Haynes admitted it might be twins and recommended she take it easy. He gave her a cone to help with the drippage. Carl was not pleased to find her wearing it at night. "This is just your way of keeping us from having intercourse," he accused.

During her repose, Carl assured Dr. Haynes that he took good care of her, rushing home from work every day to be with her. He said he'd only ever gone to the YWCA for classes to improve his English. These had been necessary for him to become a naturalized citizen (which he did that fall). Sadie reported neglect, even that he went away to fish on the weekends. She believed he was punishing her for becoming pregnant.

Dr. Haynes offered to give Sadie an abortion if she kept mum about it. Unbeknownst to her, he'd already been disbarred from one medical society for performing the procedure on others. Abortion was not officially outlawed in the state, but it was extremely dangerous in the days before antibiotics, accounting for nearly one-fifth of maternal deaths the year she gave birth. Sadie surprised him by refusing his offer. "Well, think it over," he said.

Her condition only worsened until finally, in late spring 1930, when she was about eight months along, she began to experience labor pains. She telephoned Dr. Haynes to tell him she was suffering terribly. "You're too sympathetic with yourself," he replied. She was to wait until the pains became more regular.

Around midnight on May 18, she had Carl drive her downtown to Edward W. Sparrow Hospital. When Dr. Haynes arrived, she berated him for neglecting her throughout her pregnancy. Had she not been under the influence of analgesics, she might not have been so bold.

"Keep your thoughts to yourself," he scoffed.

Carl wandered around the visitors' room until the physician came to congratulate him on the birth of twin girls. Dr. Haynes returned only a moment later to reveal that fate had actually dealt him three of a kind. He returned once more with a final update:

"You've got four of them, and none of them came up the elevator or fire escape."

Carl stood there in shock. The way he'd tell it, he was overcome with worry that his wife would die, leaving him with four poor, motherless souls. The physician would remember things differently. According to Dr. Haynes, Carl was visibly furious. The first words out of his mouth were, "What will they think my wife is—a bitch dog?" He then ran down the corridor crying, and the doctor had to chase after him. "You'll be a famous man," Dr. Haynes assured him.

The doctor's version of events would better align with that of a neighbor, who'd claim Carl came storming into her house that night crying something terrible and asking, "Why in the hell did she go and have so many kids?"

When he finally collected himself there at the hospital, Carl went into his wife's room and sat down on the bed. "It's up to you to make a good thing of it," he muttered.

Sadie had no time to fret over his feelings. She was going into an ether-induced slumber, having powered through three hours of medicated labor to hear each of her children's cries. The next day, she was preoccupied with getting the babies to latch. The smallest one, weighing only three pounds, was unable to suck, while another just licked at her breast. She felt it was a mother's duty to nurse, but eventually relented to the idea of them tube feeding. It was just as well she did, as she soon felt her limbs swelling and suspected a hemorrhage. She tried to tell Dr. Haynes, but he said not to worry. When she did develop a bleed, he scolded her for having such a notion and then making it come true.

The week the girls were born, the *Lansing State Journal* had reported on real estate, a boat race in the Grand River, and an incident of drunk driving, giving much of the front page to syndicated news. No wonder local reporters were now clamoring to see the girls. There'd been news of quadruplet births in other states, but never had the people of Lansing seen such a rare event in their own backyard.

One reporter stole inside the nursery to snap a photograph when no one was looking. Another tried to bribe a nurse to reveal their weights and lengths. Nearby dairies were fighting to supply their milk, and city officials were thinking of providing the family with a house to live for a year, after which they could pay rent or purchase the home. A few prominent businessmen in town had opened savings accounts for the girls, poets were busy crafting verses to commemorate them, and seamstresses were sewing diapers and bonnets. Rumor had it, a furniture company on the East Coast was constructing a special baby carriage to accommodate the lot.

Dr. Haynes had been right about their newfound celebrity. But what exactly it was to live in the public eye, Sadie and Carl had yet to find out.

Chapter Two

From the day they were born, the Morlok quadruplets belonged to other people. No sooner were their births announced in print than crowds began to gather outside the hospital, demanding to see the new attraction. Thousands wrote to the *Lansing State Journal* to suggest names. Sadie wanted to call them Jean, Jane, June, and Joan, but the nurses urged the new parents to give the public their say. The newspaper editors agreed this was best, establishing the *Journal* as a clearinghouse for name suggestions, gifts, and well-wishes. In the end, Dr. Haynes's ten-year-old daughter won the naming contest with her idea that each girl should share an initial with the hospital: Edna, Wilma, Sarah, and Helen for Edward W. Sparrow Hospital. This was much to the chagrin of ordinary entrants and those who'd tried to bribe Sadie with life insurance policies for the newborns.

When city officials did indeed provide a home for the family to live free of charge for one year, along with the weekly services of a health department aide, locals came round-the-clock to the house at 1023 East Saginaw Street to see the identical quadruplets, whose odds of existence were proclaimed to be one in ten million or perhaps one in twenty million. No one could say for sure. Visitors grew angry if Sadie refused them entry. As she later told NIMH researchers, they felt they should be able to peer over the children's cribs anytime they wanted. The girls' pediatrician, Dr. Horace French, suggested she charge twenty-five cents admission unless visitors had contributed to the family in some way. This made many people even more indignant. Had they not contributed to the girls' livelihood with their tax dollars? Some paid the fee only to feel cheated if the girls were sleeping or if Sadie refused to change their diapers or bathe them upon request. It was as if they considered the family to be some sort of carnival show.

Not everyone was enamored with the newborns. Some expressed disgust at the "animal-like" size of the litter, also calling Carl Morlok "atavistic." A news writer remarked that "the very rich, who could afford [multiples], seem never to have them," further linking hyper-fecundity to the lower classes. Carl's own mother agreed the situation was abhorrent, though Katherine Morlok solely faulted her daughter-in-law, whom she suspected of being unfaithful. Going back centuries, legend had it that no woman could naturally conceive more than one child from the same partner—either the divine had intervened or she'd slept around like Leda and Alcmene of Greek mythology. (Both women had fraternal twins after laying separately with their mortal husbands and the god Zeus.) "It's all very terrible," Katherine kept repeating when she saw her granddaughters for the first time. "It'd be best for them to die."

For much of human history, it *had* been common to destroy twins upon their birth. Mothers would either kill both or choose one to keep, then toss the other down a mountainside or drown it in a river. Boys were favored over girls, and healthy-looking babies over small or weak ones. Only with such infanticide could the family be protected from stigma or further bad luck. Seeming to have inherited such superstitions, the elder Mrs. Morlok was aghast when Sadie began to put the girls on display in the front window of the house.

Others disapproved of the family's getting so much for free when bread and unemployment lines were long. When Carl managed to pick up some shifts at a local forge plant, his co-workers berated him about being a scrounger. Real and imagined loafers loomed large in the public imagination, as President Herbert Hoover and his wealthy backers invoked images of lazy workers as a reason not to offer federal relief funds. Michigander Henry Ford went so far as to blame idlers for the stock market crash. "[People] wanted something for nothing," Ford told the *New York Times* in 1930. "They wanted to gamble on the Stock Exchange. They didn't want to work. The crash was a good thing; it has made them start working and thinking again."

It's possible some also resented Carl and his wife simply for keeping the girls alive when they were bound to have costly health problems. In the early decades of the century, when medical treatment of premature and congenitally diseased infants improved so much as to meaningfully increase survival rates, many people abhorred that "defectives" were now being given a chance to live. A Chicago physician named Harry Haiselden was of such a mind, controversially denying care to a baby with partial paralysis and then making a movie to promote his position. In the popular film *The Black Stork*, his fictional character alleged, "There are times when saving a life is a greater crime than taking one."

No matter their motivations, Carl's critics likely resented him even more when notoriety swept him into public office. In the fall of 1931, after a failed attempt to make moonshine in the basement with his brother, Carl ran for constable, which mostly consisted of serving court papers but would allow him to wear a police badge, carry a revolver, and hang out with real policemen. His wife had suggested the idea after speaking with the mayor about opportunities for him. He'd initially swatted it away, worried he would lose, but about a week before the election, he arranged for the printing of campaign cards bearing his and his daughters' faces. "We will appreciate your support," the cards read. He won in a landslide, sweeping thirty-seven of thirty-nine precincts.

The national media blasted the news. "Quadruplets Win Election for Daddy," declared a United Press headline. The syndicated story noted that the jobless Carl Morlok "gave five reasons why he should be constable, namely his lack of employment and his four quadruplet daughters." The Lansing mayor was elsewhere quoted as saying, "He could have run for US senate and been elected. He had no qualifications whatsoever."

It was good for the family that Carl got out of the house. From the beginning, he offered little help in caring for the infants. His only real chore was taking dirty diapers down to the basement, something he did while cursing about the "disgraceful" quantity of them. He couldn't stand the sound of the babies crying, sometimes knocking their heads together to get them to stop. Between five and six p.m. daily, when Sadie caused their most intense sobbing by putting them on the floor to strengthen their torso muscles, he'd run for the neighbors' house. There he'd sit on the back porch with his face in his hands, marveling that his wife could call them "little songbirds."

With Carl mostly useless, Sadie had no choice but to ask her mother-in-law to move in. She expected Katherine would help with warming the milk, feeding, burping, sanitizing the bottles, and other tasks whose multitude required her to abide by a very strict schedule. But the old lady proved to be more burdensome than useful, demanding that Sadie brush her hair and rebuking her for not making German dishes. She also accused Sadie of flirting with the furnace man who periodically visited the house. When Sadie became very sick from exhaustion, Carl's mother fretted that she'd gone and gotten herself pregnant again. At least Katherine developed an affection for the girls she'd initially wished death upon. She especially liked Wilma, who had an easygoing temperament.

A woman named Mrs. Wheeler proved more helpful. She kindly took on some of the laundry, sewed the girls' baptismal gowns, and entertained the quadruplets whenever the family came over to visit. But as Sadie still could not manage it all, she hired a series of girls. None lasted long—not because of the workload, but because of Carl. He impregnated one, then paid for the nineteen-year-old to have an abortion. He proposed intercourse with another, who went and ratted him out to Sadie. Another of Carl's affairs resulted in a full-term pregnancy, costing $900 (nearly $20,000 today). The child did not survive delivery.

Perhaps it was because he wanted his wife to be angelic that Carl felt compelled to go elsewhere for sex. Countless books have described this dynamic in the antebellum South, where slaveholders put their women on a pedestal and then, statues only being "nice things to look at," made trails to backyard cabins. Viewing Black women as subhuman, these men feared no reprisal from God, much less their wives. If Carl's words to Sadie are any indication, he certainly viewed some women as being so debased as to resemble beasts.

Whatever its impetus, Carl's philandering actually saved the family some money, the $900 pregnancy notwithstanding. Knowing the constable had a reputation, the girls' pediatrician invited Carl to accompany him out on the town with a few nurses with whom he was having affairs. Sadie overheard the conversation and confronted Dr. French, who promised to see the girls free of charge until they were twelve if she kept quiet. Incidentally, she had already been promised free medical care from Dr. Haynes in exchange for silence about *his* improprieties. Once, when sick with exhaustion, she'd gone into his office to have basal metabolism testing. She was all geared up with the equipment, waiting and waiting for him to come in the room. Finally she undid the apparatus and went to the adjacent room to see about some noise there. She found Dr. Haynes on the table with a nurse.

Carl's affairs and utter unwillingness to help at home weren't the worst of Sadie's worries. Before the quadruplets' second birthday, she became consumed by fears of their abduction. She saw the way some people looked at them whenever their carriage passed on the sidewalk—the way they nearly burst with desire. Her fears intensified the day a man came to the house claiming to be a friend of her husband. He claimed to be writing a chapter on the girls for a book, but Sadie couldn't help but notice how the man scanned the house, making mental note of the entrances and exits. When Carl got home, he confirmed he had no such friend. On another occasion, two men came to the house and were admitted by Carl's mother. One of the men tried to pick up one of the girls. "Folks aren't allowed to handle them," said Sadie, remembering that a local schoolyard patrol had just overheard two men talking of kidnapping the quadruplets for a ransom. She motioned for her mother-in-law to get Carl, who was out back. Carl came running into the house with his shotgun, and the two men ran out the front door. One was later caught robbing a bank.

Later in life, Sadie would point to the high-profile abduction of the Lindbergh baby as a cause of her worry. The 1932 nabbing and killing of the angelic, curly-haired twenty-month-old absolutely gripped her imagination, as it did many American parents'. In fact, the kidnapping of the beloved aviator's son was just one of an estimated three thousand such crimes to have occurred that year. The "snatch racket," as the newspapers referred to the crisis, was so severe that outlets like the *New York Times* began to include news of kidnappings alongside notable births and deaths. Affluent families hired armed chauffeurs and purchased kidnap insurance to cover the cost of any ransoms demanded of them. In some cases, they even shipped their children off to Europe for safety. The federal government waged an official War Against Kidnappers, President Roosevelt naming FBI director J. Edgar Hoover to spearhead the crusade. This created many highly dramatized manhunts without actually reducing the incidence of kidnapping—the crime was too lurid and lucrative for perpetrators to resist committing it. It wasn't until Hoover thought to have the Treasury Department trace the ransom bills' serial numbers that the number of kidnappings declined.

If Sadie was paranoid about the girls being taken, Carl was even more so. He put bolts on all the doors, erected a fence, and began to patrol the property, which they'd recently purchased from the city. He also took to sleeping with a handgun on his nightstand. One night he mistook his wife for an intruder when she was coming back to bed from the bathroom. He reached for his weapon and fired a hole through her nightgown before realizing his mistake. "I've got to be careful," he offered in half apology. "I don't want to harm you because you've got a big responsibility here to take care of these kids."

Some neighbors and relatives objected to the girls' being forbidden from leaving the yard, attending birthday parties, or having playmates—including their own cousins—over to the house. While they understood Carl and Sadie's fears, they believed the quadruplets needed to socialize. Carl invariably dismissed such concerns. "There's four of them," he'd say. "They can play together."

For the most part, the toddler girls did enjoy playing at home, though there were always strict rules for them to obey and their only toys were those gifted to them. Whenever a visitor came over, the girls were obliged to drop their things and run for their matching walnut rocking chairs, quietly moving in unison for as long as the guest stayed. They did this for their father, too, when he arrived home from work. At the first sound of his automobile in the driveway, they'd make for those chairs. Both Carl and Sadie liked the idea of their looking and acting identically, often telling people, "They're four, but they're one."

Because she'd been singled out for verbal abuse while her male siblings were thought to walk on water, Sadie was determined to raise the girls on equal footing. And by equal, she meant identical. She always dressed them in matching outfits and bows, even though this required her to stay up late mending. Some of the girls' earliest memories were of her tucking them into bed, saying prayers, and then going down the hall, where the soft hum of her sewing machine could be heard. But try as she did to synchronize every aspect of their lives, Sadie couldn't help that the girls had disparate abilities and interests. Helen, the smallest and last born, could not handle solid foods or chew as well as the others. She also continued to wet the bed after the older three were toilet-trained. Edna, the firstborn, was the most physically advanced, followed by Sarah. These two bonded together, while Wilma and Helen preferred each other.

Sadie found that Edna was generous, while Sarah hoarded everything from marbles to coffee beans. Wilma was playful but had destructive tendencies, breaking her toys for no apparent reason. Helen was totally helpless and prone to tantrums. She relied upon her sisters to tidy her belongings, going after their stowed-away stuff if they refused. Sadie resented her youngest for making life difficult for the family. Not only could Helen never keep up with the others, she behaved in very strange ways. Sometimes she would put on four pairs of panties—hers and her sisters'—to get attention. At three years of age, she began to fondle herself. Sadie suspected her truss, a contraption Helen wore to correct a double hernia, of providing stimulation. Sadie scolded her, but it was no use. Helen continued to touch herself, especially after becoming upset about something.

Some parenting manuals urged that sexual stimulation was normal, if not exactly healthy, and that nineteenth-century experts had been wrong to so aggressively repress children's impulses. Believing that masturbation, over the course of generations, led to racial decay and that they themselves were responsible for guarding white civilization, Victorian-era physicians had urged parents and teachers to prevent the habit in youth by all means necessary, including castration, circumcision, chastity belts, the application of electricity, and the blistering of the genitals. For German doctor Daniel Gottlieb Moritz ("Moritz") Schreber, immorality flourished in weak bodies, and so it was further necessary to drive it out with intense exercise, enemas, cold baths, and posture-improving orthopedic devices, to be worn day and night.

Taking the more dated view that children should be tamed into sexlessness, Sadie began to more closely surveil Helen. It did not seem to occur to her that her youngest daughter's habit might be a form of self-consolation. In addition to finding herself the last to achieve every milestone, Helen experienced the most brutal treatment at the hands of Carl, who liked his daughters exactly in order of their abilities. While Carl adored Edna, once even bringing home a tricycle for his "most beautiful" daughter, he would throw toys at Helen and call her a moron. He was especially mean to her when he'd been drinking.

The other sisters expressed their anxieties in different ways. Sarah, who was also easily upset by Carl's drunken bouts, would run for her rocking chair and move back and forth with clenched fists. Her mother later recalled, "I used to take a hold of her hands and sort of loosen them and try to be jolly with her."

Once it was Sadie who alarmed the girls by shoving her husband to the floor. Carl had wanted to take the quadruplets to the beer hall for a reelection rally, and she thought it was a bad idea. When he refused to give up the notion and seemed like he was going to strike her, she pushed him with all her might. Seeing her daughters' terrorized faces, she vowed to never again hurt him, not even in self-defense. She honored that promise, even when he forced himself on her sexually. Most of the time, though, his drinking let her off the hook. He became too inebriated to become aroused.

Sometime after these marital troubles began, Sadie ran into her old fiancé. She took the girls for X-rays at St. Lawrence Hospital, and Davenport was the technician. She felt a flood of emotions after learning he'd tried to write to her after their breakup. For whatever reason, her parents had returned all of his letters. After this encounter, Sadie found herself wandering down memory lane. The girls once came upon her crying and asked what was wrong. "One day you'll know," she told them. She never pursued an affair, and Davenport would die only a few years later.

Still, she was constantly labeled a bad wife, especially after Carl contracted a venereal disease and she opted to sleep on the floor by the side of the bed. When her mother-in-law saw the bedclothes on the floor, she suspected Sadie of being unfaithful. Sadie had no more patience for Katherine, who had now begun to run away, spit in the heat registers, stick her fingers in the food, and fake seizures. Katherine would become rigid, shake, fall from her chair, and then temporarily lose her memory. But this only ever happened when she was angry.

If Sadie ever tried to complain to her husband, or even if she voiced suicidal feelings, he said she was making too much of things. "You are just having a mad fit," he replied when she told him she thought of drowning herself in a nearby river.

Sadie didn't have the guts to go through with that plan, but she did eventually muster the courage to kick her mother-in-law out of the house. Katherine went to live with another of her sons, collapsing of heart failure a few years later.

No matter what discord plagued the Morlok house, the outside world treated the family as the American ideal. Newspapers dutifully marked the quadruplets' birthdays with heartwarming stories and photographs of prominent figures in town paying their respects. In December 1933, when a local charity invited the girls to be ambassadors for a campaign to raise funds to fight tuberculosis, the *Journal* noted how the celebrated sisters were perfectly suited for the task. They were sweet, of "sturdy build," and the picture of health. Had they been born the decade before, they might have won ribbons and been displayed at state fairs. (At the high-water mark of the eugenics era, Fitter Families contests had popularly showcased fair-skinned, blond-haired children for their contributions to the gene pool.) No one in the press seemed to notice that some of the quadruplets lagged in speech or that Helen was uninhibited—hardly the traits eugenicists desired to see. But how would they when the sisters always appeared to be smiling and Constable Morlok referred to them as his good-luck charms? "Since they came," Carl once told the local newspaper, "everything has seemed to turn out right."

The sisters' reputation only grew more sterling when Sadie enrolled them in private singing and dancing lessons and they began to perform around town. The girls sang religious songs such as "I'll Build My Castle in Heaven," along with tunes about Christopher Columbus's triumphant discovery of the New World. Seeing how much they enthralled crowds, Sadie and Carl began to take them on the road to compete in talent shows, where they earned cash prizes.

Americans' fascination with cute little girls ran deep in the 1930s, as if the nation couldn't even wait for the future mothers of the race to grow up before it put them to use. In the throes of severe economic depression, the white public yearned for a not-so-distant past—for a time before the Jazz Age had caused so many people to stray from their Puritan work ethic and find themselves in dire straits. Wanting to supplant hard-partying flappers like Zelda Fitzgerald and Clara Bow with more wholesome cultural icons, Americans pinned their hopes and dreams on dimpled, gingham-wearing toddlers like Shirley Temple, who charmed sailors by shimmying up the aisle of an airplane as she sang about a "Good Ship Lollipop." What better persona to distract from news of stock market crashes, dust storms, and orphan trains than a baby vamp who batted her eyelashes and sang cheerily? Even President Franklin Delano Roosevelt recognized the symbolic significance of this particular child star, remarking in 1934, "It is a splendid thing that for just 15 cents, an American can go to a movie and look at the smiling face of a baby and forget his troubles."

While the singing and dancing competitions brought both accolades and a small income (not nearly as much as Carl would pretend), they also increased tension between Helen and her siblings. The littlest sister struggled to memorize the choreography, often crying during rehearsals. This frustrated Edna, Wilma, and Sarah, who complained to their mother about Helen's inabilities. Sadie made sure the girls always put on a good face before going onstage, never permitting anyone to see signs of strife. She felt that little girls should always be pleasant, there being enough wretchedness in the world. They should especially stand up straight and sparkle when singing about their country.

The gulf between the Morloks' carefully curated public image and their lived dysfunction might only have widened were it not for the girls' matriculation. In 1935, just before they took their "sister act" on the road, the foursome entered kindergarten at a local public school, giving outsiders glimpses of the anxieties beginning to grip them. This might have seemed a good change, but in flying the coop, they were more vulnerable to strangers' gazes. Between school and show, they were *always* onstage, always bearing the brunt of others' varied desires.

Chapter Three

The year before the Morlok sisters went to school, lightning struck the small, lakeside town of Corbeil, part of the Canadian province of Ontario. There a family welcomed a brood even more improbable than Carl and Sadie's. The Dionne quintuplets were the first known lot of five ever to survive infancy, and for that they, too, became public property.

It all started when the Dionne parents couldn't afford to pay for the extremely underweight babies' expensive care. The Red Cross assumed their custody, assuring the parents this unusual arrangement was only temporary. When the girls could thrive outside incubators, they would be returned. Less than one year later, and with much public support, the Ontario government passed the Dionne Quintuplet Guardianship Act, making them wards of the Crown. For the next nine years, the sisters lived in a specially built facility fitted with living quarters, a classroom, and an outdoor playground. The public could view them through a one-way screen and then browse one of the many nearby souvenir shops. Three million people visited "Quintland," which far surpassed Niagara Falls as the most popular destination in the country. Clark Gable, Jimmy Stewart, Bette Davis, and Amelia Earhart were just a few of the famous Americans who traveled to behold the girls whose images were licensed to promote products ranging from Lysol to Quaker Oats. (The proceeds from these ventures went toward the costs of running the facility, along with the hotel dinners of visiting psychologists.)

When news of the Dionne births first reached her, Sadie claimed to be relieved to share the spotlight. Then, as the government took possession of the girls, she expressed shock and sympathy for the parents who had to go through hospital administrators to interact with the girls or request any changes to their regimens. Her remarks served as fodder for those wishing to disparage Canada and glorify the freedom-loving United States, where, it was said, such a thing could never happen. Privately, however, Sadie believed the town had laid claim to her own children, if not as egregiously.

When the quadruplets went to school in 1935, she and Carl took great pains to shield them. On their first day of kindergarten at Oak Park Elementary, only reporters were permitted to document the occasion. Onlookers were told not to approach the family as they walked the few blocks to school. Like marching soldiers, the quadruplets moved as a single, inviolable unit. All in identical clothing, with the exception of differently colored bows to assist their teachers in distinguishing them.

Upon arriving at school, reporters asked what they wanted to do first. They whispered among themselves, and then Edna replied that they'd like to write their names on the blackboard. Chalk was furnished, and bulbs flashed as they performed this feat. Some classmates looked on with envy. Their resentment would only grow as teachers gave the girls special treatment, standing near them on the playground and allowing them to enter the building immediately upon arriving in the morning, while everyone else waited for the bell. Both measures were to reduce the risk of kidnapping, which seemed especially high after someone telephoned Sadie to say she should not expect Sarah after school—she would be going to a certain classmate's house. The classmate's mother denied ever making such a call.

Aside from begrudging their VIP status, students disdained the girls simply because Helen cried for much of the day and her sisters were unable to console her. They called Helen "crybaby" and the rest of the group the "dumb Morloks." The boys were far meaner than the girls, a few of whom took pity on the quadruplets. If any of the girl classmates ever dared to speak up, the boys would harass them, too. Edna, Wilma, and Sarah came to feel even more ashamed of their little sister. Sarah would later reminisce, "We were in class enjoying ourselves, and it got so that I would wonder sometimes if I could get through what I was doing before Helen started crying. It was embarrassing."

After a while, Helen began to retaliate against the bullies, hitting them and throwing their coats on the floor to make room for her own. It wasn't until the first grade that she could get through the day without shedding any tears. Even then she'd bawl when the bell rang for final dismissal. "It was just sort of a release," her first-grade teacher told NIMH researchers. "She'd been holding it together all day." According to this educator, the youngest Morlok also had an endearing habit of reaching out to pat her whenever she was upset. "Everybody who came in contact with Helen couldn't help but love her."

None of the bad experiences ever made it into print. Reporters preferred more fanciful accounts of the quadruplets' school lives, writing, "Gallantry is magnified... boys spring to their aid" and "little playmates squeeze to sit beside them." When Sadie and Carl remarked on the girls' above-average intelligence but their teachers reported they were "slow, normal little girls," reporters went with the parents' perspective. They also downplayed the Morloks' protectiveness, which some school personnel were beginning to describe as a form of "parental suffocation."

At first, teachers wondered if it was because they lived on a busy highway that the quadruplets were never allowed to ride bikes after school. Then they wondered if their parents didn't approve of their being with boys. But none were ever able to gain Sadie's confidence, as she refused to become involved with committees like the parent-teacher association. They'd later learn that Carl forbade her from taking on any responsibilities that might jeopardize her commitment at home. If homeschooling had been established as a respectable alternative to public education, Carl probably would have desired it for his daughters, but it would be another few decades before the public really began to take such an alternative seriously.

Over the next few years, teachers took it upon themselves to expand the girls' social lives. After learning that the sisters had never attended a birthday party, one decided to throw a picnic during school hours. Much to this woman's disappointment, the Morloks just ran around by themselves "like young lambs let loose in a field." Another teacher arranged for a field trip to a local factory, but was unable to persuade Carl and Sadie to permit their daughters to go. Still another dismissed students from class for them to attend a parade and then write an essay about it. Carl stayed home from work that day and prepared a special dish for the family—something he never did. The quadruplets never made it to the parade.

It also bothered some teachers that the sisters used the plural voice. If asked questions, they answered with "we." Their mother, too, spoke this way, referring to "their cough" even when only one or two were ill. She also referred to the girls as "her only child."

Sadie once explained herself by saying that, since their birth, she could only see or think in groups of four.

Beginning in first grade, teachers made a point to separate the girls in the classroom. This was all right with Edna and Sarah, who were more confident and thought by their parents to be more academically capable, despite there being little difference in all the quadruplets' grades in those early years. Sarah took pride in having the most social connections. This led to some mild rivalry with Edna, who, according to Sarah, "got everything first." (Not only was Edna the firstborn, she was the first to lose a tooth, smile, and say a word.) Mostly, though, these two sisters bonded over their perceived superiority. When they began to share a bedroom, they whispered about Helen. Neither wanted to be classified with her. Their father urged that Edna, being the eldest, was responsible for Helen. It was her job to see that Helen never ran away, something that would be a huge embarrassment to the family. Helen took advantage of this situation, demanding that Edna do her favors like tote her belongings to and from school. One day she insisted that Edna hold her coat, and Edna refused. Helen began to drag the coat on the ground, knowing their mother would be upset by the dirt. Edna sighed and took the garment.

In her grade school years, Helen also grew more cunning at home. She once went into Sadie's sewing corner and cut up cloth that was to be used for a set of outfits. Sadie retaliated by stitching the scraps together into a dress and then making Helen wear it to school. There was also the time Helen told a teacher that Sadie didn't feed her. The teacher had remarked on her comparatively small size, and Helen replied that she was denied meals while her sisters got to eat until they were full. The school officials called Sadie to the school to explain herself. Outraged by her daughter's fabrications, Sadie demanded Helen come in and tell the truth.

It was plain to Edna, Wilma, and Sarah that Sadie disdained Helen, even blaming her for things that were not her fault. She was a "scapegoat in everything," Sarah later explained. But an adult Sarah would also wonder if, at least at first, Sadie's dislike didn't lend itself to a deeper love. "While all the blame went on Helen, way down there was an understanding in a protective way between Helen and my mother…I think she was trying to guide Helen in her ways of thinking. There was a closeness." The tender feelings only faded when Helen continued to masturbate, and "Mother seemed to turn against her."

Carl and Sadie often found Helen lying awake at night with her legs crossed and her hands gripping the side of the bed as she moved rhythmically. They were deeply disturbed to have such a passionate child. Carl asked the teachers to look for evidence of her sex play during school hours. The teachers did so, but saw nothing alarming. Carl then demanded to know if her sisters were aware of anything untoward. She did wiggle a lot in her seat, they reluctantly offered, adding that she went to the bathroom often. If the elder three resented Helen, they also felt protective of her. None wanted to see Carl's fury come down upon her.

When the girls were in second grade, Sadie began to suspect the school janitor of fondling Helen. In her mind, this would explain why Helen's nasty habit had never resolved. The other sisters reported that this man—the janitor—would often meet Helen in the hallway and ask, "How's my little girl?" He also had pet names for her, though not for any of them. He once picked Helen up, bounced her in his arms, and remarked on the truss that she wore. Mrs. Morlok observed such behavior with her own eyes when the man once stopped by the house to say hello to the girls. She'd gone to another room, then returned to find him with Helen straddled over his knee. She immediately asked him to leave.

Sadie approached Helen's teacher with her concerns about the janitor but was dismissed. "He only takes to her in a friendly way because she is so vulnerable," said the teacher, recalling a time the janitor had found Helen crying in the hallway and returned her to class. In her mind, this incident seemed to prove his pure intentions. "Well, Helen doesn't like to be picked up," Sadie replied. The janitor was not to touch her anymore.

Perhaps it was an entrenched, though emphatically disavowed, pedophilic gaze that prevented Helen's schoolteacher from imagining any impropriety. By the late 1930s, children had been thoroughly sexualized in print media and on the big screen. Norman Rockwell was painting youngsters in their undergarments for the *Saturday Evening Post*, and the Morton's Salt Girl debuted darker lips and a higher hemline. The transformation of it-girl Shirley Temple offers the most vivid case in point. The Tinseltown toddler began her screen career in 1932 wiggle-dancing in *War Babies*, a film about an exotic dancer who catches the attention of two soldiers (played by other tots) in a café. By the close of the decade, she was a top-grossing box-office star with various films in which she danced and flirted with actual adult men, including a Black man in *The Little Colonel* (1935). In a review of *Wee Willie Winkie* (1937) for his magazine *Night and Day*, novelist Graham Greene observed that her real-life admirers—mostly middle-aged men and clergymen—rather liked "the sight of her well-shaped and desirable little body, packed with enormous vitality."

Indeed, J. Edgar Hoover liked that little body enough to sit it on his knee when he had a private audience with Temple. So did hundreds of others, leading one of Temple's biographers to call her a "connoisseur" of laps. These encounters might have been innocent enough, but in the years following Greene's review, other men took far greater liberties. One studio executive unzipped his trousers and exposed himself to a twelve-year-old Temple. Another used a remote switch to lock the door of his office and then tried to grope the teenager. A producer attempted to seduce her by saying, "Look, I'm going to be a big executive. We're going to have to get along." When she protested, he boasted, "Sex is like a glass of water. You get thirsty, you drink. You want sex, you have it."

In 1937, the producer of *Wee Willie Winkie*, Twentieth Century-Fox, expressed outrage over Greene's remarks, joining with Temple's guardians to sue him and his magazine for libel. Greene's magazine folded, and he left for Mexico, allegedly to avoid criminal prosecution. But he was no pervert, according to present-day scholars; he was merely exposing the dynamics of Temple's fame. In the words of Susan Jennings Lantz, Temple's "body of work (to say nothing of her corporal body)" had indeed begun a "subtle process of deconstructing the image of an asexual innocent childhood and building...a sexuality that was decidedly infantile in nature." In showcasing smooth-skinned, doe-eyed youngsters like Temple, Hollywood could give droopy-spirited audiences a blank screen on which to project all their fears and desires. This might have been lost on President Roosevelt when he described Temple as a morale-boosting national treasure, but it was not lost on moviemaker D. W. Griffith, who wrote to Temple's producer in response to her dancing with a Black man in *The Little Colonel*, "There is nothing, absolutely nothing, calculated to raise the goose-flesh on the back of an audience more than that of a white girl in relation to Negroes."

By the time Sadie approached Helen's teacher about the janitor's possible misdeeds, mainstream culture had effectively normalized the sexualization of children. Which would explain why no one seemed to bat an eye when Paramount Pictures produced a one-minute reel of the quadruplets showing them eating breakfast, washing at the sink, polishing their father's police badge, and then—just before the clip ended—beginning to undo the buttons of their clothes. Along with other short reels of curious people, this was screened in theaters across the country before the showing of a feature film.

But only young and respectable individuals could enjoy children. Elderly white men, known homosexuals, and Black men remained suspect—and the janitor was none of these. Such figures were widely depicted either as "sexual psychopaths" (elderly and gay men) or beasts (Black men) who needed to be removed from polite society before they corrupted children. Drawing upon Freudian notions that sexual development began in infanthood, public officials reasoned that aged, senile individuals often resorted to an earlier stage of development, finding themselves attracted to children and no more able to control their impulses than those they lusted over. In the case of homosexuals, the problem was that normal development had not occurred, often because men had lacked a conventional father-figure with whom to identify or been subjected to a smothering mother. Never learning healthy masculinity, these individuals, too, related to and abused the young.

Sexual psychopath laws offered a solution. These authorized law enforcement to arrest questionable persons and surrender them to asylums until psychiatrists deemed them safe, in some cases by castrating them. The Morloks' home state of Michigan was the first of twenty-six states to pass such laws at the behest of authorities like Hoover, who called for a "War on the Sex Criminal" like his War on Kidnapping. With kidnappings on the decline, Hoover needed a new high-profile cause to justify his bureau, and this particular project may have appealed because it provided cover for his own alleged homosexuality. In the words of Charles E. Morris, III, "a man so dedicated to the scourge of degenerates certainly could not be one." Across the nation, local police worked to round up suspected perverts. Carl may have had a hand in apprehending some such deviants, as he often rode along with officers.

As for Black men—they were beyond rehabilitation, theirs not being a case of arrested development. White psychiatry declared that humans' maturation literally repeated the evolutionary path of their ancestors—from primitive to civilized—and that the Black race had not yet evolved to an advanced state. Popular culture promoted this view by endlessly portraying Black men as savages who threatened white girls and women, requiring racist vigilantes or their partners in law enforcement to forcefully intervene. Griffith's 1915 film *The Birth of a Nation* famously depicted a southern belle jumping off a cliff to evade a Black man (a white actor in blackface), prompting members of the Ku Klux Klan to chase down and kill her assailant. The blockbuster movie succeeded in reviving the terrorist organization first begun in the nineteenth century. Over the next few decades, Klansmen and other racial terrorists lynched thousands of Black men and even boys for such offenses as looking white women in the eye, knocking on white women's doors, or addressing them with less formality than observers deemed appropriate. Contrary to popular belief, these lynchings were not confined to the South. Nor were efforts to hide racial terror behind sexual innocence.

Following the separate murders of three local girls in 1937, the *New York Daily News* filled its pages with photographs that variously emphasized their purity (wearing a confirmation dress, playing with dolls, and frolicking at the beach). One victim was nine-year-old Brooklynite Einer Sporrer, who was part of a pro-Nazi German American bund (political club). Sporrer's funeral has been described as a "pageant to innocence," heavily featuring her white-wearing, choir-singing playmates. It implicitly reminded girls everywhere that guarding their chastity was their most important responsibility, while also making a larger statement about what kind of people embodied virtue. Never mind that thirty-five members of Sporrer's bund unit were seen extending their arms in Nazi salute outside the church and then again at her gravesite.

Such was the world in which the Morlok sisters found themselves. It was a world that professed to be protecting children from violent predators, but that sanctioned racial hate and largely ignored sexual abuse occurring in homes, churches, and schools at the hands of familiar people.

It wasn't only the janitor whose potentially assaultive behavior adults ignored. Others got away with ogling and touching the plaited-hair, ribbon-wearing girls, often in situations where the girls were performing their goodness. Sarah would later say of being backstage in their quaint dance costumes, made to resemble Temple's, "People would molest us in some way, trying to pull our dresses and prowl around and shove us." Her mother said not to worry—these people were only envious of their success.

Partly because of the constant groping, the girls preferred lessons to showtime. "It was always their happiest time of the week," their singing and dance teachers would later tell NIMH researchers, adding that their father seldom attended these sessions. According to the two instructors, Carl had a habit of starting arguments about religion and politics. The dance teacher, Virgiline Simmons, thought him a bully, who refused to permit either his children or his wife to make any friends. At least he seemed to take pride in the girls' celebrity. Carl would walk around venues and tell strangers he had sired the famous set. When one master of ceremonies called him and Sadie onstage to take a bow, he happily obliged. On this occasion, the girls had opened for a minstrel show, in which a cast of adults "played Negro" aboard a riverboat named *Robert E. Lee.*

When the sisters were seven, a child talent agent proposed that Sadie move them to New York, where they could compete full-time. Another man in the child entertainment industry suggested Hollywood, claiming to have connections to establish them there. Sadie did consider these prospects, especially as they offered a chance to get away from Carl without actually divorcing him. She'd previously consulted a lawyer about leaving him when the girls were six, but he'd found out and promised to be better. (As it happened, the lawyer had gone to Carl and persuaded him that he'd never find a woman as godly, clean, and punctual as Sadie, so he shouldn't take her for granted.) After this, Carl had begun to eavesdrop on her telephone conversations and read her outgoing mail. He didn't want her to send any letters to relatives that were the slightest bit unfavorable to him. Sadie rarely saw her family members anymore, as Carl complained whenever they stayed overnight and would not permit her to visit Ohio. He did not even budge when her mother died, asking, "What good would you do being there now?"

Carl's drinking had become more excessive as well. He often put the girls in danger by driving under the influence to their out-of-town shows, while a police escort followed behind. Sadie suspected him of consuming eight to fourteen bottles of beer a day. She couldn't say for sure as he often drank at taverns with his police buddies and then refused to discuss the matter, even when she asked for the sake of his insulin dosing. Sadie needed to give him shots that correlated with his glucose intake. Too little insulin and his blood turned acidic; too much and he could have seizures or lose consciousness. Carl decided to give himself the shots so she would get off his back.

Since the girls' infancy, he'd become more violent, pushing Sadie around and threatening to kill people who had slighted him in any way. One day Sadie wondered if he had taken a life. He came home drunk and appeared as though he'd been in a brawl. He anxiously paced while she inquired about his whereabouts. "Don't worry about it!" he snapped. Three days later, a detective came by the house in connection with a body found in the river. (It's unclear if this official was familiar to Carl.) The corpse belonged to the second husband of his former sister-in-law, Loretta. She and Carl's brother Bill had divorced a few years before. The detective reported that a witness claimed to have seen three men on the bridge the night the victim drowned. Did Carl know anything about this?

Sadie watched as her husband fumbled through the interview then, upon the man's departure, as he stormed out the back door and cried. A few weeks later, he went down to the detective's office and offered to help locate Loretta in another state. "How would you know where she is?" the detective asked. Carl didn't answer. Instead he said something about how he'd been the one to advise his brother to get the divorce—he'd known that woman was trouble.

The authorities never got to the bottom of the suspicious drowning, but Sadie assumed Carl's guilt. He would become agitated and make threats in his sleep, once even outright declaring that he had killed someone. When she tried to rouse him from his slumber to explain himself, he said, "Maybe I did once."

He also boasted of roughing up people on the job, leading her to wonder what other trouble he got into. But when it came to violence against perceived ne'er-do-wells, Lansing authorities tended to look the other way. Only a few years before, the police had refused to investigate when the home of a Black family burned to the ground, even trying to charge the patriarch, a Baptist preacher named Earl Little, with arson. The Littles had been living in a whites-only neighborhood, riling members of the Black Legion, a midwestern offshoot of the Klan. Nor did police investigate when

Little was struck by a streetcar, dying later at Sparrow Hospital, where the quadruplets had been born. The family again believed the legion responsible.

Partly because Carl spoke so belligerently about people, Sadie was inclined to believe him when he threatened, "If you ever leave me, I will find you wherever you go and kill you." But she did not confide in anyone about this threat or any of his other abuse. Instead she devoted herself to maintaining appearances, mostly by restricting press coverage to special occasions and always setting the editorial tone with sentiment or humor. Her husband and children learned to be prescriptive with their tone, too. Once when the family went to a local department store for the girls to meet Santa Claus, Carl made light of the girls' request for drums and bugles: "Four drums going at once—I don't know." Only a few days later, when asked if they had a message for the Dionne quintuplets, the quadruplets whispered among themselves and answered, "Could we say Merry Christmas to them?" News writers dutifully reported such charming remarks.

Sadie kept scrapbooks with all the press coverage and recital programs, which the girls routinely perused, along with an album of news clippings of their idol, Temple. She knew her daughters took great pride in their accomplishments and the attention they received. They were especially in need of affirmation when Helen had to be held back in school and Sadie, still focused on equality, made all four repeat the grade. But there may have been another reason for the scrapbooks, as one of the NIMH researchers later surmised: They provided "a kind of looking glass in which the girls could gaze at their own reflections and learn something of who and what they were expected to be."

Unlike the Dionne sisters, who had no sense of the external world or the unusualness of their situation, the quadruplets were keenly attuned to the public's perception of them. They further knew that their parents' contentment depended upon their playing their parts. This meant controlling their tempers and smiling through tears. Keeping family secrets and learning not to recoil at strangers' touch. Guarding certain aspects of themselves, while offering others up for mass consumption.

In retrospect, it would be easy for some to see how injurious this life was—how it was only a matter of time before the girls conditioned to be public darlings went stark raving mad. Yet beyond noting how Carl's overbearing ways impeded their social lives, no one around the Morloks said a word about their burdens. Nor did anyone appear to notice when things turned more sinister at home. People kept snapping photographs of the little house on East Saginaw Street, and important figures continued to visit. A relative of the Dionne quintuplets even stopped by to pay her respects. No matter what was going on behind closed doors, the view from outside always remained rosy. The looking glass was also a kaleidoscope—it could transform the darkest of scenes into multicolor wonders.

Chapter Four

David Rosenthal was born in Harlem in 1916, nine years after his parents, both European Jews, arrived at Ellis Island with little more than a few personal effects. Like many first-generation Americans of the day, he had an austere childhood. His parents could not afford lessons in Hebrew, so he never even achieved his bar mitzvah. In Brooklyn, where the family moved when he was four, he lacked even a bed to sleep on, pushing chairs together for a makeshift one. He spent his days playing ball in the streets, running footraces, and reading under the kitchen table, his "bed" having been disassembled for the day. He devoured dime novels, along with books on science, history, and philosophy. Early on his family pegged him the studious one, deciding he should stay in school even when tragedy struck.

When Rosenthal was twelve, his father died of suspected tuberculosis. The family was too poor for a doctor, so no one could say for sure what caused the man to collapse after several weeks of coughing and belabored breathing. Both his older brothers dropped out of school to support the family, while he stayed the course. He'd already skipped a few grades and mastered several languages, and everyone wanted to see how far he could go. Even then people knew he was going to be someone.

At fifteen, Rosenthal graduated high school and went to work as a jeweler's apprentice, earning enough money to enroll part-time at one of New York's city colleges. After his mother remarried and the family moved to Ohio, he transferred to a university there. Then came the draft.

On September 16, 1940, President Roosevelt signed into law the Selective Training and Service Act, which required all men between twenty-one and thirty-five years of age to register for service. In 1942, after the United States officially entered World War II, Rosenthal was one of ten million other registrants to be formally inducted into the military. Were it not for this call of service, he may never have set down the path that would eventually cross with that of the quadruplets.

Not long after getting his uniform, Rosenthal boarded a commandeered luxury liner. No one could say exactly where he and his new peers were headed in the vessel, whose fancy carpets and decor bore strange witness to its heyday. Nor did they understand why they were part of no convoy and instead totally exposed to German submarines. He would later learn and record in his diary that this particular ship could actually outspeed any enemy warship. This detail certainly would have comforted a fellow soldier named Bakrak, who'd make a lasting impression on Rosenthal, standing on deck "waiting for the torpedo to hit and ready to heave himself into the sea."

The days went by quickly for the precocious kid from Brooklyn. He loved to observe the patterns of the ship's wake and the dolphins swimming in the distance. Spending so many hours above deck himself, he became friendly with Bakrak. After landing in North Africa and training for combat, all the men made their way to

Naples, where the Allies had overtaken an Italian hospital. The day they arrived, they were ordered to dig foxholes for themselves in a nearby camp. Rosenthal carved only a foot into the earth before his hands began to blister and he sat down to rest. He wondered if his commanders were merely trying to scare them—he hadn't seen any signs of enemy craft. Bakrak seemed to have no such doubts. Only a few feet away, Rosenthal documented, this GI "was digging like mad."

Around twilight, someone screamed "air raid," and the diligent ones made for their holes. Those who'd slacked ran to the hospital for protection. Rosenthal panicked for a moment, then hopped into his "pipsqueak of a hole." He must have made a ridiculous sight with most of his body aboveground, but from his crouch he watched a show like nothing he'd ever seen before. The planes sprayed bullets and dropped colorful flares to illuminate the entire harbor. There were "great upsurgings of light" and "streaks of glowing red, green, blue and yellow." Searchlights crisscrossed the terrain to the music of the artillery. He'd never felt so alive.

At one point, over the earsplitting sounds, he could hear Bakrak screaming. He went over to the trembling man, who could not manage to look up from his hole. Still feeling exhilarated, he squatted down and began to narrate the scene. Strangely, it seemed to put the man at ease. One could call it Rosenthal's first therapeutic encounter.

When the raid ended, the men crawled out of the ground and began to babble about what had occurred. They walked around and marveled at the long, jagged pieces of heavy steel that could have turned any one of them into confetti. It wasn't until the next morning when they got to the hospital that they realized there'd been casualties.

As this hospital was away from the front, most days and nights were not quite so perilous. Still, with all the roving trucks and northbound aircraft, there was a perpetual sense that something was happening or about to happen. The GIs complained about the lack of plumbing and real playing cards, but most were grateful for a tent to sleep in and cigarettes to light as they told and listened to stories—endless stories. In the city, the soldiers encountered spirited locals, many of whom had given blood, money, and land to fight the fascists. War was "a world that had its own fascinations," and Rosenthal couldn't help but feel that he "might really down deep miss it when it came to an end."

Before it did, he was assigned to assist a neuropsychiatrist, witnessing wonders of a different order. One soldier after another came into the hospital with the loss of some bodily function, though no tissue damage or evident maladies. "Men with two good legs suddenly couldn't walk... Some couldn't see, or hear, or talk, or remember." In therapy, all were made anew. Others got wind of their recoveries and came to be healed.

Rosenthal couldn't help but revere this neuropsychiatrist, who professed to hate Nazis as much as he loved psychoanalysis. He eagerly accompanied "Captain B" on his morning rounds, watching as the man gently but firmly commanded men to walk. Some couldn't. They'd fall, and onlookers who didn't know better would think the captain cruel for mocking an injured GI. But after a few days, these men would take steps, knowing their problems were in their heads. Rosenthal would remember these times as "the glory days of psychiatric healing."

In early 1945, the high-flying bombers began to taper off, and he suspected the brutal war was coming to its creeping end. Sure enough, Germany surrendered in May, following Hitler's suicide. Some soldiers began to fret about civilian life, but not him. Having become so very fascinated by the psyches of his fellow men, especially following shell shock, he knew his next calling.

Back in the States, he finished his undergraduate work at the University of Akron in Ohio. Then he was off to George Washington University for a master's degree in psychology and, after that, the University of Chicago for a PhD in the same field. Psychoanalysis dominated the study and treatment of mental disorder, though in mutated form and often going by the term *psychotherapy*. The discipline had largely abandoned Freud's sexual focus, with analysts now conceiving of mental dysfunction in terms of familial dysfunction. According to medical historian Anne Harrington, most of these neo-Freudians were interested in "how to live an authentic life of love and work...And virtually all were attracted to the idea that psychotherapy could and should be emotionally nurturing rather than aloof."

That America took to psychoanalysis at all must have been a great shock to Freud. When Clark University president and psychologist G. Stanley Hall invited him to lecture in the States in 1908, he was initially reluctant to accept the offer, thinking a visit futile. In his mind, Americans were materialistic and prudish—even the most educated circles would not give him a fair shake once they discovered the sexual core of his theories. But he eventually relented, perceiving an opportunity to spread his cause, which was then little known. In a series of lectures delivered in German in September 1909 at Clark, Freud laid out his theories of the human psyche. He introduced the concept of the unconscious, defined hysteria as the product of reminiscences, explained how neuroses could be traced to early-childhood sexual impressions, and touted his talking cure. It was the first time he neatly tied all of his philosophies and therapeutic innovations into one program, which made an immediate impression on such esteemed audience members as psychologist William James and anarchist Emma Goldman. Following the lectures' English publication, the wider public was hooked.

While some did indeed rebuff psychoanalysis as a "filthy examination" into patients' past sexual lives, many recognized Freud's extraordinary insights into the human psyche. Advertisers soon began to incorporate his principles into their marketing, and psychiatrists trained in the methods of analysis to offer this form of treatment to those with means. For those who couldn't afford to hop on the couch or who wanted to protect their children from developing hang-ups, popular magazines like *Good Housekeeping*, *Everybody's*, and *TIME* identified common defense mechanisms and their latent meanings, while bestsellers like Dr. Benjamin Spock's 1946 *The Common Sense Book of Baby and Child Care* instructed parents on ways to rear psychologically healthy offspring.

If by midcentury, talk therapy had been adapted for the worried masses, Rosenthal remained committed to the deeply disturbed. The war had shown him how profoundly trauma could afflict people—and what marvelous transformations talking could bring about. At a time when journalists were beginning to expose the horrors of asylum medicine, talk therapy may have seemed all the more urgent. The press reported that state institutions built in the nineteenth century had dramatically devolved. If once they had provided a bucolic setting for people to roam gardens and find their way back to reason, they were now overpopulated with society's unwanted. Doctors performed grueling treatments like insulin coma, shock therapy, and lobotomy. How, critics asked, could a nation permit these abuses and claim to be any different from Nazi Germany?

Freudian psychology may also have appealed to Rosenthal because of its seeming secularity. Even though the US had played an enormous role in ending the Holocaust and its people identified as defenders of freedom, its institutions were not exactly welcoming of viewpoints that were not white Protestant. But here was a discipline that challenged the Christian worldview and that was populated by European Jews who'd been forced to emigrate before or during the war, when Hitler forbade mention of Freud. By some accounts, it was precisely Freud's antipathy toward Christianity that had shaped his enterprise. Both of Freud's parents had been subjected to severe anti-Semitism in nineteenth-century Europe, where the Roman Catholic Church had long incited violence against Jews with different myths about them: They killed Christ, worshipped Satan, purposely spread the plague, controlled the banks, and routinely preyed upon Christian children, using their blood to make Passover matzo and thereby ritually reenacting the crucifixion. (The Roman Empire executed Jesus.) Resenting how Christians had persecuted his people and also identifying more as a secular Jew, Freud determined to replace religious doctrine with the "science" of psychoanalysis. It's not hard to imagine why a nonbeliever like Rosenthal would take to this discipline, even if he did not share Freud's view of religion as a form of neurosis—and even if he made room for Christianity in other facets of life.

While he was doing fieldwork for his master's at a veterans' hospital in Perry Point, Maryland, he met a social worker named Marcia Kensinger. She had it all: beauty, smarts, and wit. The only problem was that she was Presbyterian. For this reason, Rosenthal's mother, now living in Washington, DC, did not approve when the two became engaged. He'd never forget her first words to his soon-to-be wife: "I never thought he'd do this to me." Marcia's parents in Iowa were also apprehensive about the arrangement. To avoid conflict, the two got married by a justice of the peace shortly after David began his doctoral studies. They welcomed their first daughter, Laura, the following year.

Marcia did convert to Judaism for her mother-in-law's sake, but refused to give up Christmas, which turned out to be the family's only religious practice. Their son, Scott, who was born in 1954, shortly after Rosenthal began a post-doctoral research fellowship at Johns Hopkins University, would not step foot in a synagogue until college.

At the prestigious Baltimore university's Henry Phipps Psychiatric Clinic, Rosenthal studied the interactions between patient and psychotherapist. Curious to know if improvement correlated with an adoption of the therapist's moral values, he developed a sixty-item rubric to assess parties' attitudes toward sex, aggression, and authority (the main areas of behavior around which psychological conflicts tended to arise). According to a subsequently published paper, which applied this rubric and a few others to twelve patients and their therapists, patients who moved toward therapists' value systems did indeed fare better, while those who moved further away were unimproved or even worse at the end of treatment. This led Rosenthal to propose that, even when trying to avoid doing so, therapists communicated their values in subtle and unintended ways. As these values tended to be less absolutist than patients', the improvement could be due to greater harmony between the patient's moralizing superego and the rationalizing ego. It could also be that the more individuals could accept others, the more they could accept themselves. Such suggestions evidence Rosenthal's commitment to both Freudian principles and a relational view of mental illness.

He was soon appointed to a professorship, exploring ways to

strengthen psychotherapy, such as by optimizing the group therapy setting. Schizophrenics, whom he had studied for his doctoral dissertation, seemed particularly in need of psychotherapy. At the time, their mental disturbances were being reconceived as the product of mother love gone wrong. Both the nineteenth-century German psychiatrist who'd identified schizophrenia—Emil Kraepelin, who'd called it *dementia praecox*, meaning "early dementia"—and the Swiss psychiatrist Eugen Bleuler, who'd renamed it, were sure that schizophrenia had an internal origin. But the 1930s saw a few studies linking the illness to dysfunctional mothering. Then a German Jewish refugee analyst working at the Chestnut Lodge sanitarium in Rockville, Maryland, threw open the door to this line of inquiry. In 1940, Frieda Fromm-Reichmann used the term *schizophrenogenic mother* to describe mothers who bore healthy children and then drove them mad with a severe, dictatorial manner. The petite analyst known for her grandmotherly facade refined the concept in a 1948 publication. Here Fromm-Reichmann suggested that it was actually a mixture of hostility and overprotection that shattered psyches. Such "early warp and rejection" in infancy and childhood caused schizophrenics to be "painfully distrustful and resentful of other people." Psychotic behaviors were a means for them to make sense of the confusing communications at home.

Fromm-Reichmann was not solely focused on mothers as the source of mental disturbance. In fact, her 1948 essay was primarily about ways to strengthen the therapeutic relationship. Nevertheless the schizophrenogenic mother theory would become her legacy. Almost as soon as she first articulated it, researchers sought to prove her right, some asking if there was a connection between this personality type and the Nazis who'd risen to power in Germany. One research team even developed a scale to test mothers of schizophrenics for their fascist traits. Such rushes to judgment mistook her intention: stirring hope and compassion for patients. Whereas Freud had declared schizophrenics incapable of "transferring" their feelings onto the analyst (and thus therapeutically irredeemable), Fromm-Reichmann believed even the most disturbed schizophrenics could be reached in analysis. And whereas Freud literally looked down upon his patients on the couch, she saw hers face-to-face, even sitting in some of their urine to convey that she did not view herself as superior. She also accepted patients' feces to show that she wholly accepted them. In her mind, those in crisis only needed to be properly loved and nurtured to begin healing.

Rosenthal would engage the notion of the schizophrenogenic mother in his later writing. For now, his work on schizophrenia expanded to include an investigation of a muscle relaxant's effects on patients with the diagnosis. Of all the afflictions he encountered, he remained most fascinated by schizophrenia, the so-called heartland of psychiatry, and it was this interest that prompted an old colleague to contact him in 1954 about an extraordinary case on his hands. Dr. Leonard Himler claimed to have in his care a set of twenty-four-year-old identical quadruplets, all of whom had been diagnosed as schizophrenic. Rosenthal must have alerted researchers at NIMH or referred Dr. Himler directly to these people, as, soon after, NIMH dispatched a psychiatrist to the quadruplets' home to see the sisters for himself.

Chances were, Rosenthal knew that the scientific director at NIMH, Seymour Kety, was planning to investigate the roles of genetics and environment in the development of schizophrenia. Kety was a neuroscientist who suspected that the brain held clues to genetics, and he was going to look at twins to confirm it. Twin studies had long been cited as evidence of the heritability of schizophrenia, as they showed higher concordance rates (both twins diagnosed) in monozygotic twins, who shared the same genetic code, than dizygotic ones. But this finding did not satisfy those who believed that parents—namely mothers—"taught" their children to be crazy. These critics noted that monozygotic twins also shared more of their environment than dizygotic twins. The twin studies were dismissed for the additional reason that their pioneers—psychiatrist Ernst Rüdin and his mentee Franz Josef Kallmann—had worked with the Third Reich, and it was unpopular to think about genetic factors in the immediate postwar years. (Rüdin had actually served as the architect of the Nazi sterilization program; Kallmann, who was partly Jewish, had advised the Third Reich to examine schizophrenics' relatives for the purpose of sterilizing "nonaffected carriers" before fleeing to America and becoming involved with the eugenics movement there.) It seems that Kety was less bothered by any nefarious affiliation than by the studies' shoddiness. He was certain it was possible to separate the effects of nature and nurture, as well as to "build a bridge across the big chasm between basic knowledge of the brain and mental illness."

If there was any institution equipped to build such a bridge, it was NIMH. The newly formed institute was headed by a neo-Freudian, Robert Felix, but also a component of the National Institutes of Health (NIH), which meant that it was closely connected to organizations focused on diseases, such as cancer. At a time when the specialties of psychiatry and neurology were growing apart, NIMH's leaders agreed that neither social nor biomedical research should be conducted in a vacuum. To build a world where fewer Americans developed and suffered from costly mental health problems, as Felix had promised Congress in order for the social experiment to come to fruition, they needed to think holistically. The National Mental Health Act of 1946, which called for the institute's establishment, had further provided $10 million (about $164 million today) for the construction of a building, which was then supplemented by $62 million (about one billion dollars today) from other institutes to create a state-of-the-art Clinical Center for all the branches to share. There really was nowhere in the world better positioned to undertake the sophisticated twin studies that Kety conceived.

Not long after Rosenthal referred the quadruplets' case, a research psychologist named Morris Parloff, who had been at Hopkins before going to NIMH, suggested that Kety bring Rosenthal on board for the studies. At first, the director of the adult psychology lab, Dave Shakow, rebuffed the idea. Shakow had been one of Rosenthal's professors at the University of Chicago, and he claimed to have been unimpressed by his dissertation. Parloff assured Shakow that Rosenthal was doing good work at Hopkins and urged that the two meet for lunch. They did, and Rosenthal dazzled his former professor, accepting a job offer shortly thereafter. As was common practice during the McCarthy Era, he first had to prove he was not a communist by answering extensive questions about his politics and pledging his loyalty to the US.

Rosenthal then moved his family of four into his mother's place and began work, as he and his wife looked for a home close to the NIH campus. House-hunting took some time, as many neighborhoods had covenants forbidding the sale of homes to Jewish, Black, and Italian families. Realtors would hang up on Marcia after hearing her last name. Finally, the family was able to get into a neighborhood in Bethesda developed by real estate mogul Ted Lerner and known for its preponderance of government scientists. The three Rosenthal children—another daughter, Amy, would come along in 1958—would grow up thinking everyone's father worked at NIH.

Rosenthal quickly fell into a rhythm, walking to work and returning home in time for a five thirty dinner, after which he'd call his mother then turn on the television or read a Thomas Wolfe novel. He and Marcia bought a used piano, spending Sunday afternoons writing music for it. A post at NIMH did not a rich man make, but Rosenthal was clearly moving up in the world, far removed from his days of sleeping on chairs and one step closer to the publication that would catapult his career.

Chapter Five

If there was one fear that relentlessly gripped Carl Morlok, it was that of his loved ones' animality. Years after first calling the mother of his children a "bitch dog," Carl continued to suspect Sadie of being unfaithful—of having insatiable desires. And as his girls began to mature, he sniffed for something feral in them, too.

Whenever his daughters were around boys of the same age, which outside of school was seldom, he would watch them closely. A flushed cheek was enough for him to interrupt their play and announce it was time to go home. He didn't even relax in private. Spurred by his deceased mother's superstition that leftover food should be browned deeply in order for their hogs to breed, he accused his daughters of "trying to get stimulation" if they ate so much as a darkly toasted slice of bread.

The latter was too far-fetched even for someone with Sadie's sensibilities, but Carl managed to persuade his wife of his other convictions. For instance: A cousin of his had gone crazy from masturbating. This may have been easier for Sadie to accept because religious tracts still trafficked in Victorian pseudoscience, warning that, beyond corrupting the soul, "self-pollution" could lead to mental dullness, muscular atrophy, or even death. As Sadie wanted her daughters to be spiritually and physically strong, she supported Carl's extreme measures to curb the habit in Helen.

At eleven, the youngest Morlok was still hopelessly addicted to touching herself and seemed to have turned some of her sisters on to sex play. After once catching her in the act, Carl and Sadie confronted the others about their own behavior. Wilma confessed to having "done things a little." Edna threw up, giving her parents the impression that she, too, was implicated. Sarah did not seem to understand what they were asking. After conferring with each other, the parents decided to make an example of Helen. Sadie swabbed her clitoris with carbolic acid, as the other three looked on in terror. She explained that the skin-corrosive antiseptic would make the bad flesh melt away. The acid caused a superficial burn, which eventually healed.

A week later, at the recommendation of the family pediatrician, Dr. French, Sadie took Helen to see a child psychiatrist about the problem. This expert claimed to find no underlying disease to account for Helen's masturbation and assured Sadie that she would eventually grow out of it. He did, however, express worry about Helen's "listlessness" and "lack of vitality," which had become evident when she sat motionless in play therapy. Perhaps Sadie should try to ease the pressure on her. This would help Helen to gain confidence and better relate to others, in turn giving her the gumption to do things for herself.

A social worker at the office formally recorded other misgivings about Sadie. After interviewing her, this professional noted that the "self-assured" woman "quickly made her identity known as the mother of the Morlok quadruplets," seeming to enjoy her renown and even the occasion that had brought her in. While Sadie had remarked several times that it "pained her" to talk about Helen's behavior, she didn't betray the slightest anguish in her tone or facial expression. If anything, she seemed rather giddy.

These notes reveal a personality in contrast with her husband and the person she was purported to be. Whereas Carl seemed to be discomfited by the simple fact of the quadruplets, fearing their quantity evidenced low breeding, Sadie appeared only to take pride in having birthed four all at once. Perhaps because she came from somewhat better means, she was not inclined to think of herself or her children as "white trash." But Helen's masturbation *was* something that would push them beyond the pale of middle-class respectability. As she told the social worker, she couldn't understand how a girl who went to church could engage in such behavior. Yet sincerely unnerved as Sadie was about Helen's sex play, she couldn't help but delight in discussing something so taboo. Puritanism and prurience went hand in hand, giving credence to latter-century French philosopher Michel Foucault's idea that one way to have sex was to talk about it.

Sadie didn't talk long, at least not with this set of professionals. Soon after the visit, she telephoned the clinic to say she would handle Helen herself. Irritated, the psychiatrist recorded that she was a "very inflexible and controlling kind of person" who refused to listen to authority and who therefore could not be part of the solution. She appeared to be expecting "something quite magical" with regard to Helen, and when this didn't occur, she did not return.

That the psychiatrist solely suspected Sadie as the source of her daughter's psychological troubles may be due not only to his meeting solely with her, but also to his profession's longstanding denial of male abuse—something arguably abetted by Freud. The father of psychoanalysis had begun his career with a foundational theory of sexual trauma. After spending the early 1890s analyzing cases of hysteria with his colleague Josef Breuer, he claimed to have found a "great clinical secret": An astonishing number of (female) hysterics seemed to have had a prepubescent sexual experience combined with revulsion and fright. Freud's patients hadn't reported seduction in plain words, but rather related dreams and images that seemed to him to involve it. When he suggested abuse, some denied any memories of such. Still, the link between early-childhood sexual assault and adult hysteria appeared so firm to him that he adopted the motto, "What has been done to you, poor child?" But not long after presenting his seduction theory at an 1896 conference, he began to retreat from it. Most hysterics who relayed sexual impressions were just expressing fantasies, he decided. He couldn't say where their fantasies came from, but he was certain they revealed some deep internal truth that the patient wished to repress. This belief—that fantasies signified some unspeakable truth—led to his Oedipal theory, which asserted that children desired sex with the parent of the opposite sex and hated the same-sexed parent.

A growing discourse of maternal failure may also have influenced Helen's psychiatrist. Frieda Fromm-Reichmann had by now introduced her theory of the schizophrenogenic mother, and psychiatrists were shifting focus from castrating fathers (the primary figures in classical Freudian psychoanalysis) toward overprotective and icy mothers. Were it not for this climate, Helen's psychiatrist might have surmised that however problematic Sadie seemed, she might not be the only perpetrator of harm.

In later interviews with NIMH researchers, Sadie contradicted the psychiatrist's stated reason for her never returning to the clinic. She claimed she overheard Helen telling Wilma that the doctor said it was all right if children touched themselves. She was furious that he would plant such a debased idea in her daughter's head. She was also angry at Dr. French for recommending him.

In their continued effort to get their daughters on the straight and narrow, Sadie and Carl moved the quadruplets' beds down to the dining room so they could keep an eye on them until they fell asleep. They also began to frighten the girls with claims about the physical consequences of masturbation. Children who fondled themselves did not grow and became very stupid in school, they warned, knowing that Helen's small size and academic struggles would make the point stick. Carl also told of his gone-mad cousin, which seemed to particularly disturb Wilma. She wanted to know, would she become mentally ill from what she'd done?

Helen asked no questions. Interpreting this as stubbornness, Carl and Sadie did not bother to give her another chance to change her ways. According to an adult Sarah, they immediately devised their next steps: "They had remedies in mind like a certain type of berry that is prickly... They thought of using a hot iron and almost got in the process of such things. My father discussed using a knife." There was also talk about a kind of juice that, when applied to the vagina, would make friction uncomfortable. While Carl and Sadie never resorted to any of these particular methods, they "would whip her. They would dunk her head in water when they felt she was not acting how she ought to, mostly when she would cry." It was usually Carl who yearned to punish Helen and Sadie who executed his whims. "He seemed to want to let her do the job." Sometimes, though, it was Carl who would hold Helen facedown in the basin, then count to ten as her arms flailed in every direction.

No one ever asked what happened to Helen in these moments—if she prayed, if she left her body. There was an unspoken understanding among the others that she should not have to relive them, and Helen had never been very good at articulating her feelings. Silence prevailed among family friends, as well. One remarked about Helen's bruises, prompting Sadie to reply that Helen had fallen down the stairs. Nothing more was said. Maybe this woman felt that pressing the issue would only make things worse for the littlest Morlok. Maybe, instead, she was satisfied by the answer, as domestic abuse—like sexual abuse within the home—was not on many minds, at least not for longer than it took to push the troublesome idea away. The public could rest comfortably in ignorance because the medical profession routinely covered for physical abusers. Just as doctors fabricated the idea that children could acquire venereal diseases from towels and toilet seats, they reached for alternative reasons for the incidence of unexplained broken bones. Papers published in medical journals in the 1940s show physicians speculating that a mysterious new children's disease was appearing on the scene, which would explain why so many kids presented at hospitals with injuries.

As time went on, Carl became so determined to catch his youngest daughter doing wrong and then beat her for it that he took to standing outside the bathroom. If he thought she had been in there too long, he'd barge in. He must have been satisfied the day his wife found twelve-year-old Helen engaged in mutual masturbation with Wilma, proving she was as deranged and corruptive as he believed. He certainly didn't doubt Wilma when she claimed it was Helen's idea. Nor did Sadie, who took both girls to see Dr. Haynes, the man who had delivered the quadruplets, about the incident. Dr. Haynes gave them a salve to apply and demanded they douche with cold water before bed. The masturbation had to stop, he urged. The girls' frequent bed-wetting was because of it.

When it didn't stop, Dr. Haynes suggested circumcision, which was commonly performed on girls thought to be "over-sexed" and thus prone to mix with other races. By cutting the clitoris, he claimed, he could remove their urges. Hearing this proposal, Wilma burst into tears and promised to behave. Whatever Helen was feeling, she again kept to herself. The girls went under the knife shortly thereafter.

The day of the operation, Wilma was hysterical, pleading for another chance. This enraged Dr. Haynes, who jerked her around the surgical table just for asking. He used such force preparing her for the procedure that she was black and blue by the time he carved into her. But it was Helen whom the man really loathed. As he later told NIMH investigators, she was unsightly and coarse—not the least bit girly like the others. She was "skinny and sweaty and moist" and impossible to impress with the usual tactics of shame or fear. She was a "genuine antagonistic," who frankly "didn't care who was told about [the masturbation] or who knew about it." Not even physical punishment made an impact—it "didn't hurt her." Never in all his years of practice had he seen such a "lone wolf."

Much to the consternation of Edna and Sarah, who'd only been vaguely told what was going on, Wilma and Helen remained in the hospital for several days. During this time, both broke their stitches, indicating they'd once more reached between their legs. Wilma was the first to tear the threads, prompting the physician to threaten to fix her for good. If she didn't gain ahold of herself, Dr. Haynes warned, he'd "cut out all her flesh." The man Sadie had once caught sleeping with a nurse evidently had no patience for wayward girls, much less any desire to hear their side of the story.

Upon the girls' release, Haynes ordered Carl and Sadie to tie their hands to the bed and give them sedatives to keep them from thrashing and wailing. The parents were to do this for a full month. That first night, Carl and Sadie did exactly as they were told, also forbidding Edna and Sarah from seeing their sisters. Still they found Helen in the morning with red marks on her hips. She'd been trying to get at herself with her elbows, and not because her stitches itched.

Why did Helen persist to the point of injury? What was the nature of the ache inside her? Was it a longing to be touched or something more fraught?

Experts had long disagreed about the impetus for compulsive masturbation, some offering quite outlandish theories. German psychiatrist Richard Freiherr von Krafft-Ebing once argued that a degenerative constitution, rather than any external factor, was to blame. Not unlike Carl's mother, Michigan physician and eugenicist John Harvey Kellogg, director of the Battle Creek Sanitarium, believed "exciting and irritating foods" to be a cause, urging that children eat bland foods like the cornflakes cereal he and his brother had invented for asylum patients with indigestion. Kellogg also blamed "wicked nurses," writing in 1881, "Incredible as it seems…it is not an uncommon habit for nurses to quiet small children by handling or titillating their genital organs. They find this a speedy means of quieting them, and resort to it regardless or ignorant of the consequences." While formulating his seduction theory in the 1890s, Freud, too, suggested that early sexual experiences could be the genesis of compulsion, though he did not singularly blame servant women who came into the home. Early assault by a father or other male figure could arouse a child's eroticism and also cause hysteria, making masturbation a form of fantasy and repression. (Later accepting that infants had the "germs of sexual impulses," he decided that masturbation addicts were stuck in a narcissistic stage of development.)

Could it be that the school janitor *had* violated Helen and she was perpetually reenacting the abuse? Sadie was the only one to suspect the janitor's influence, though not exactly in terms of trauma. She believed he had encouraged vice in Helen, and then Helen had encouraged vice in Wilma. There was little room in her mind for complex psychological motivations. If her daughters masturbated, it was because they liked it.

Was it possible that Helen and Wilma were also rebelling against their parents? Sadie may have thought so after she overheard them laughing about her not knowing anything about masturbation. They described her as some kind of dunce who could not accept that it was normal, even after being told so by the expert. Two months after their surgery, Sadie brought them back to Dr. Haynes to recount their mockery. "I can tell you right now, they are institution cases," Haynes replied. He then telephoned the psychiatry clinic to convey his disapproval of the psychiatrist's handling of the situation.

Sadie doesn't seem to have seriously considered sending her daughters to an asylum. Perhaps the incident with the psychiatrist made her feel that doctors could not be trusted. The prospect of Wilma and Helen talking to strangers about their home life may also have dissuaded her. Sadie once let slip to one of the girls' schoolteachers that Carl was afraid they'd tell family secrets if they grew close with anyone outside the clan. And that was before they'd begun to lash Helen with a belt and plunge her head underwater.

In lieu of committing Wilma and Helen, Sadie decided simply to separate them at night. When she caught Helen trying to get back into bed with Wilma in the middle of the night, she moved Helen to a cot in her and Carl's bedroom, where she remained until they left for Bethesda more than a decade later. There were no more recorded visits to Dr. Haynes, who soon moved upstate to work for a public asylum and become a preacher, offering his surgical services to church members for a reduced fee. Sadie would still catch Wilma and Helen masturbating, though usually not together.

Other worries began to take the foreground. Helen was falling even further behind in school, and the other three had grown more despondent. In addition to witnessing trouble at home, they'd been forced to give up their singing and dancing. It pained Sadie to have them drop out, but she'd simply become too exhausted to keep up the duties of stage mother. After 226 shows, they now only performed in the occasional variety program at school. In November 1942, soon after Helen and Wilma's surgeries, she suffered chest pain that required her own hospitalization.

Her family doctor told her she'd had an angina attack, though a cardiologist later performed an electrocardiogram, which came back normal. In his view, there was no certain diagnosis. Sadie was bedridden for some weeks, requiring someone to tend to her and help around the house. Edna, Wilma, and Sarah agreed to take turns so Helen didn't have to miss any school. Sadie indicated that she didn't want her youngest nearby anyway.

With both their parents becoming more hostile toward Helen, the elder three showed more love for her. Once when a boy was teasing Helen on the playground, Edna nailed him to the ground and began to pound him. Sarah had to coax her away before any teachers noticed. She herself tried to help Helen at the piano so she would have something to be good at, and Wilma always put on a jubilant mood for her. Sarah later related that Wilma never complained much anyway, but when Helen was feeling down, "it was sunshine all the time."

It seems that all of the girls could have used a break from the limelight, but it was not to be even after their retirement from show business. As it was preceded by the nation's formal entry into World War II, the press had already improvised a new public role for Lansing's most distinguished citizens: wartime patriots. Newspapers printed photographs of the quadruplets variously "doing their bit for Uncle Sam," such as by purchasing war stamps at the Sears Roebuck store, participating in the Clean Plate Club campaign to conserve prepared food, and joining their schoolmates in scrap drives. Accompanying stories embellished their work as cheerer-uppers. "In our city, so long under the pall of dark, gloomy skies, there is at least one place where there is no gloom today," a *State Journal* contributor wrote of the family's home on the morning of the girls' twelfth birthday. "Somewhere the sun is shining...Somewhere the children play." By all accounts, the quadruplets were fighters of fascism, not victims of another iteration of it, here at home.

In private, Carl was rooting for the Third Reich. The father of the quadruplets could not read the newspaper without expressing his awe of the führer. Once Germany won the war, he hoped, America would be purged of its own waste humanity. Sometimes he made his feelings known when the family was out in public, compelling his wife to shush him. "You're American now," Sadie would scold. "They'll deport us if you talk like that." The quadruplets, for their part, would turn red and look to see that no one had heard him.

Having made the sisters icons of innocence, journalists could not easily have acknowledged Carl's virulent hate, if they did know about it and conventions permitted such reporting. Their hands somehow forced, they probably would have resorted to euphemism, as the *Lansing State Journal* did when it described fifteen thousand robed Klansmen marching through town as a "colorful parade." Nor could members of the press have easily reckoned with Carl's sexual appetites, which would help to explain why they seemed to sidestep the open secret of his extramarital affairs. One writer reported on the constable's recovery from a "blood infection" that was almost certainly a flare-up of his venereal disease or even a new one. Around this time, Carl had been visiting another woman in town and staying until two in the morning. This woman actually visited the house while Carl was out to ask Sadie if she would permit him to stay with her for longer periods of time. Surely Sadie was too busy to miss him. "Are you having an affair?" Sadie responded. The woman's face flushed. Carl continued to visit her, parking his car on the street for all to see.

The innocence beat also demanded that writers shield the family from criticism that they were charity cases—because no one was wholesome who depended upon others, as Carl so keenly understood. During the war, when rationing and absent income-earners forced many families to tighten their belts, reporters gave space for the Morloks to proclaim that they didn't "receive any special consideration" from local businesses or public agencies. "I hope nobody believes that because we buy four identical dresses or pairs of shoes, we get a discount," Sadie once told a correspondent for the Associated Press, adding elsewhere that she and her husband would never stand for such extensive government aid as the Dionne quintuplets received.

Rather than noting that the family was actually drawing upon a college fund begun for the girls by Lansing's Business and Professional Women's Club, reporters made a point to emphasize the Morloks' humbler-than-most lives. "Their pleasures and most of their fun is at home," wrote a *Detroit Free Press* contributor. "One thinks a bit before sending four little girls to the movies, and one doesn't say, 'let's have ice-cream soda,' to four little girls at the spur of the moment." Another writer added, "In case you are under any misapprehensions, quadruplets are a strain on the exchequer as well as the nerves." In this story, an interviewed Sadie made sure to clarify that she did not view her children as a burden. She believed all children were a blessing and that the word *burden* should not be used to describe anyone unless that person were an atheist or an outlaw.

If only society agreed, Lansing welfare workers would not have routinely stormed the home of Louise Little, the widow of the preacher terrorized by the Black Legion, and looked with disgust upon her and her seven children, who were now receiving a small mother's pension. Whereas city officials had worked to see that all of the quadruplets' needs were met, welfare workers denied Little's request for glasses for one of her children, paid her a smaller stipend than they paid white mothers, and disapproved of her driving a car when public transportation was available. When she became pregnant by a man she was seeing, a county judge removed her children from the home, committed her to a mental asylum in Kalamazoo, and then turned his attention to her kids, one of whom had been caught stealing from a grocery store. A physician diagnosed her as having "a paranoid condition, probably dementia praecox," citing her extreme suspicion of people and her claims of being discriminated against.

Even before they themselves were found to be paranoid, and though they never met Little, the Morlok sisters were knotted to this woman and her children. They were cast as the Littles' foils in a great tragic drama. If the Littles' home was over-surveilled, the Morloks' home was under-surveilled. And if the Little children were forced into early adulthood, the Morlok children were suspended in Neverland.

Members of the press largely avoided grappling with Edna, Wilma, Sarah, and Helen's entry into teenage-hood in 1943. Around their birthday, the *Detroit Free Press* advertised a Sunday feature on the thirteen-year-olds under the title "The Four Little Morloks and How They Grew," a riff on Margaret Sidney's popular children's series, *Five Little Peppers and How They Grew* (1881–1916). In the pursuant story, the writer noted the Morlok teenagers' long legs, more honey-colored hair, and bluer eyes, but gave more attention to the childlike delight he surmised they'd take in beholding their birthday cake. Meanwhile, an *Escanaba Daily Press* writer imagined the four teenagers "merrily skipping" home after school to celebrate their big day. It was as if they hadn't aged at all.

But for all the media's diligence in ignoring the fact of the quadruplets' aging, it was Carl and Sadie who were the most determined to keep the sisters young. In contrast with Little, who taught her children to resist society-assigned roles, they played the game. Their efforts to keep up the fantasy of youth would shock NIMH researchers, as well as Edna and Sarah, who quickly found that their good behavior would no longer protect them from their parents' strange compulsions. After years of watching from the sidelines, the favored two daughters began to experience mistreatment firsthand, and all four came to cower like children, if no longer resembling them in physique. The sisters took to eating with their heads down and crying under their covers, as they learned that what happened to some teenagers in the daytime could be far more terrifying than the things little ones heard go bump in the night.

Chapter Six

They were too perfect, just too good," one of the quadruplets' junior high teachers once reminisced about them. "In class, they usually sat just like mice."

If, in retrospect, this teacher ever discerned something nefarious about the foursome's mannequin-like presence, it was not the case during their years of school attendance. When the foursome entered Pattengill Junior High in 1943, this teacher and others only believed, as grade school teachers had before them, that the Morloks were a little smothered by their parents. No one surmised what dark feelings lay behind their smiles. Nor did the two scientists who published a research article on the family that fall, on their life outcomes as multiples. Writing for the *Journal of Heredity*, Iva Gardner and H. H. Newman reported that the quadruplets were thriving and attributed this to their near-normal lives. In contrast with the Dionne quintuplets, wrote Gardner and Newman, these girls were not "wards of a government and therefore somehow sacred."

Thinking the sisters too uniform, teachers and school administrators delighted when one of the quadruplets' personalities or even naughtiness broke through the family facade. Take the time the school office began getting phone calls about a popular girl in the sisters' class. Sally Murphy was trouble, the unnamed caller alleged. After a few weeks, an administrator managed to trace one of the calls to an empty office in the building. There was Helen Morlok with a receiver in hand.

"It tickled us," a teacher recalled. "We were just so pleased that Helen could be that devilish." No one punished the girl for the incident, and there is no record of her parents having been alerted about it. Chances were, they would not have been so amused.

Now that the quadruplets were teenagers, school personnel had no patience for their dressing all alike or as two sets of twins, as was becoming more common. (With the war making it harder for Sadie to find four matching outfits, she'd buy one set for Edna and Sarah, and another for Wilma and Helen.) It seemed to staff that girls on the brink of womanhood should present as individuals—not the identical dolls the newspapers portrayed them to be. But the sisters appeared to take offense to any suggestions that they look more distinct. When asked if she and Edna would at least part their hair differently, Sarah privately joked that she ought to come to school in blackface. Perhaps, deep down, the girl once made to open for minstrel performers intuited that blackness was exactly the opposite of that which society expected her to embody.

Administrators only ever disapproved of differentiating the quadruplets if it was Helen being singled out. Once, when Sadie asked for Helen to be separated from the others to improve her focus, the school principal suspected that she was actually trying to punish her youngest. Still, this official obliged, and Helen began to find excuses to leave her classroom to go find her dear Wilma.

There was only one teacher who did not like the quadruplets. She would scoff at them and say, "I would have to die to get my picture in the paper. You girls got it on account of being born."

She once told Sadie they were "freaks" and so she should plan for them to "stay on the domestic side." Sadie told her daughters not to pay her any mind.

The quadruplets were too busy trying to survive their male peers' aggressions to care much what she thought anyway. Boys would knock their books out of their hands, call them names, and throw orange peels and silverware at them in the cafeteria. "We had to watch our step every minute," Sarah later recalled. "I would be walking down the stairway and I'd have to watch that somebody didn't just come up behind me and push me down because they didn't like us, that we were four." More than once at home, they found the wooden steps pulled away from the porch, as if people wanted them to walk off it and fall. On one occasion, they discovered a pitchfork lodged in the front door. Their experiences stood in sharp contrast with newspaper headlines about servicemen flooding the home with love notes. They did receive some gushing letters from soldiers, though not nearly as many as the media purported. One can only wonder how it felt to enthrall these strangers while disgusting acquaintances. Were they confused by the contradictory emotions they stirred in people? Or was it something more like shame that gripped them, as a result of not living up to expectations?

The mistreatment at school became so bad that Sadie intervened. She suggested the principal make an announcement over the loudspeaker about there being no tolerance for bullying. The principal had another idea. Why not allow the quadruplets to attend school dances or join a club? Making connections outside the classroom would go a long way. "We are self-sufficient," Sadie replied. "The girls do not need that."

She and Carl also rebuffed their church minister when he encouraged the quadruplets to join the youth group, claiming that a co-ed group would be "a demoralizing factor for them." They even pulled the sisters out of confirmation classes after learning that the instructor allowed time for the students to socialize. This instructor came by the house wanting to know what the problem was. After hearing their concerns, he suggested rescheduling the recess for the end of the sessions so they could pick them up before it began. Carl and Sadie relented, and the girls returned.

When the time came for the sisters' junior high graduation banquet and it was indicated they could not attend, one of their public school teachers similarly intervened. Showing up unannounced, the teacher asked why the sisters couldn't go. Sadie explained that she and her husband couldn't afford formal dresses for four. Well then, the teacher responded, she could make two gowns, and Sadie could make two. Cornered, Mother Morlok agreed to think it over. Soon afterward the sisters reported that the Lansing Ladies' Aid Society was going to provide them with evening wear. Sadie must have seemed stubborn, appealing to this organization rather than accepting the teacher's help, but all that mattered was that the quadruplets had permission to go to the dinner.

As the big night approached, Carl badgered his daughters with notions of what could go wrong. He was sure someone—probably Helen—would step on her dress and tear it. Still, none of the sisters could be dissuaded from attending. They'd never looked forward to anything so much. Everyone agreed Wilma should do their hair, as she enjoyed playing beauty parlor and was the most adept at pinning curls.

That night their class was scheduled to entertain right before dessert was served. Just as the sisters concluded their performance, drawing applause, a figure appeared in the back of the room. It was Carl, come to say their mother was very sick in the hospital. Distraught, the girls begged to be taken to see her. They grabbed their things and piled into the car, soon realizing that their father was not driving in the direction of the hospital. They looked among themselves, and one mustered the courage to ask what was going on. Carl just kept focused on the road. Only after pulling into the driveway and killing the engine did he offer any words. "You've been there late enough."

Edna ran upstairs crying. Carl proposed ice cream for the other three, seeing as they'd missed dessert. They refused. In that case, he said, it was time for bed. It was only half past eight.

Edna often complained to their mother about incidents like this, but Sadie said there was nothing she could do. Though she'd later try to distance herself from her husband's officious ways, she was actually the one to communicate most rules on his behalf, especially those pertaining to boys. An exception was the subject of marriage. Carl himself made clear there was to be no chatter about it. They were "not dry behind the ears yet," and he did not believe in young marriages—they inclined people to a larger family size. He himself had been one of ten children (one of whom died young), and he was not proud of this fact. Should any of his daughters become engaged before the age of forty, he would not take her to the altar.

The Morlok parents' guardedness kept potential suitors away once the quadruplets did begin to attract some positive attention from male peers. So did the sheer number of sisters. One of their classmates at Eastern High School would confess to NIMH researchers, "The thought entered my mind a couple of times to ask one of the girls to go out. What held me back was the fact that there were four of them." Another peer who lived nearby and sometimes walked Edna home would relate that he was "a little afraid to ask one out, because they were quads and because [their mother seemed] like a matron cracking a whip." When Edna made the first move and asked if he'd like to escort one of them to junior prom, he was startled. He fumbled for a moment, then claimed that financial difficulties prevented him from attending. Edna was very kind about this, he'd go on to tell researchers. She said they probably wouldn't go for the same reason, but both knew it was really because the sisters were not permitted to attend social functions. Not even football games, which their parents could've supervised.

Girlfriends were now permitted to come over to the house, though Carl often chased them away. He once blew his top to learn that one had a boyfriend. Because of incidents like this, their socializing remained mostly confined to school. A homeroom classmate would later relate, "I wasn't close to them outside of homeroom, but I felt very close to them there. It was a strange kind of friendship."

It pained Edna, Wilma, Sarah, and Helen to be kept like babies in a crib when they could peek through the window and see neighbors of the same age going off with chums. But these disappointments paled in comparison with the trauma of being infantilized in an altogether different way. When the sisters began to blossom, their parents refused to accept the course of nature.

Sarah would never forget the time she approached her mother about her sprouting breasts. Sadie gasped in horror. "What happened in school that made you get these bumps?" she asked, insisting that Sarah answer her at once. Sarah racked her brain, eventually remembering that she had walked into the coat rack a few days before. She didn't think she'd hit her chest, though. That was all Sadie needed to hear. She ran to the medicine cabinet for salve to reduce the swellings. Needless to say, the remedy did nothing to flatten the "bumps."

When Sarah got her period shortly before the quadruplets'

fourteenth birthday, she didn't even try going to her mother for guidance for fear of upsetting her. "I felt so guilty," she later reminisced. "I tried to figure everything out for myself. It was so hush-hush."

If any of the quadruplets ever dared to ask questions about sex, Sadie answered evasively or not at all, in that way taking after her own mother. It didn't matter if she'd been the one to stir their curiosity. Once Sadie threatened her daughters with pregnancy if they ever went out with boys. Sarah thought about this for a moment. "I don't know the role of the father in producing the baby," she admitted. Sadie pretended not to hear her.

Another time Edna confessed that a boy had put his arm around her and she saw a bulge in his pants. She wanted to know if it was true that a girl couldn't get pregnant from her first time having intercourse. She'd heard rumors to that effect. Sadie assured her that she could indeed become pregnant, while refusing to explain what sex was.

Years later, the Morlok matriarch would defend her approach, saying, "If they knew too much, there was no way of knowing how much trouble they would get into." This was the attitude of many of the era's opponents of sex education, who viewed even the most rudimentary human anatomy lessons as part of a communist plot to mongrelize the races. Advocates countered that knowledge was necessary for the young to learn to control their appetites and protect the race. Thanks to the influence of racial purists like the now-deceased G. Stanley Hall, high school health textbooks largely urged students to mind the color line.

Wilma expressed her own opposition to sex education on a school survey about dating attitudes, which ended up in NIMH investigators' hands. (Whether the others took the same survey is unknown.) Wilma also aligned with her parents in finding ethnic and religious compatibility to be very important in a relationship. Maybe she genuinely held these views. Or maybe she was too terrorized by her parents to disagree even privately. Sadie claimed good daughters went along with their parents without ever questioning. According to an elder Sarah, their mother felt especially entitled to their devotion "after all she'd done for them."

Sadie was hardly the only parent to dictate her children's morality and politics, especially in an era when fears of civilizational decline ran deep. What distinguished her was the lengths she took to isolate the quadruplets from external influence during school years when even more sheltered individuals tended to enjoy greater social and intellectual freedom. And, of course, her repeated failure to protect her children from the monster at home.

During this time, Carl began slacking at work so as to lurk around the house. At first, it was only a few commitments he neglected to be present when the quadruplets were home. Then he began to have his partner do more and more of his job, saying he couldn't trust anyone "in this day and age"—he had to supervise his daughters.

Supervising included molesting. Carl began to grope the quadruplets' breasts and buttocks, claiming he needed to gauge how they'd react on dates when older. He no longer permitted them any privacy, standing in the doorway as they changed in and out of their nightgowns. If any of them ever tried to turn away from his gaze, he would barge in and confront her for the slight. And if anyone ever closed the door to the bathroom, he'd accuse her of slamming it in his face. Not even the changing of sanitary pads garnered the quadruplets any privacy. He'd say, "You're just like everybody else in the world so don't think you have anything special." Sadie never intervened. She simply made a point not to go away for extended periods of time in case her husband tried to take things further. It was as if everything short of rape was all right with her.

Later pressed to explain Carl's behavior, she'd claim pride that her daughters had resisted his advances. In her mind, it was proof that they were "good girls."

His authority unchecked and his daughters now approaching their high school graduation, Carl decided they shouldn't marry at all—not even when they were forty. It would be better for them to work. If they all lived together, they could keep the home free of debt and also support him when he became too old and sick to work.

Now in his mid-fifties, Carl was seriously declining, and he was not ashamed to use this fact to demand his daughters' innocence and maintain his influence over them. According to NIMH researchers, "the implication was always present that if they did date, they would involve themselves sexually and become pregnant," thereby pushing him to death. Sadie seemed to think, however, that Carl's diabetes or alcoholism would suffice to do him in. She often spoke of his one day dropping dead, mostly to prepare herself for the possibility. She wondered if they could convert the upstairs into an apartment for lease. Sometimes Carl went along with this scenario, saying his death was imminent. When he was drunk, he became more threatening. He'd vow to shoot himself or even the whole family unless he got his way.

Edna was incredibly disturbed by such talk. Sometimes she would go to her room to cry about their father dying. Even though he put his hands all over her, and even though she quarreled with him over his many rules, she didn't want to lose him. According to Sarah, Edna never pushed back too hard about any of his rules because she didn't want to lose the privileges that came with being his favorite. She liked being paid compliments and spoken to in a softer voice than he used with the others. Perhaps she also savored their relationship for approximating the romantic ones she was denied. In Sarah's words, Carl treated Edna like a second spouse: "He wanted all of her attention, in some respects the kind of attention he would get from another wife, not sexually of course, but just in other ways: time, compliments, devotion." By this point, these were about the only intimacies Carl could withstand, impotence being among his ailments.

Sarah also fretted about Carl dying, though for different reasons. She had become more religious while studying the Book of Revelation in confirmation class. The descriptions of the end of days, combined with the Exodus commandment to "honor thy father and mother," created intense pressure in her. She felt she had to be good to prevent catastrophe striking her family.

Carl rather enjoyed these two sisters' distress. Sometimes Sadie would come home to find him pretending to be fatally ill. She only needed to announce that she was phoning the doctor to get him to perk up. Knowing Sarah was more religiously inclined, he also stirred her fears by saying that if anyone got killed, she would be the cause. In God's eyes, she was a sinful creature who deserved every punishment that came to her. Even though Sarah was so obedient, he frequently accused her of disregarding the faith he and Sadie had worked so hard to instill in her. Both she and Edna began to let the idea of college slip from their minds.

Helen and Wilma did not seem bothered by the idea of their father's mortality, perhaps because his treatment of them had long been more severe. They carried other burdens. Helen was becoming more inert, prompting her mother to take her back to the psychiatry clinic. (Sadie must have been very worried to return to the expert who'd drawn her wrath.) During these visits, Helen refused to share her thoughts or even engage in normal conversation.

Asked if she enjoyed any activities such as swimming, she replied, "Oh, we don't swim." Asked what classes she was taking in school, she replied, "Oh, just what we are taking now." Mostly the now-eleventh-grader played checkers with herself while the psychiatrist looked on. At one appointment, she sat in silence for nearly thirty minutes until finally offering, "I think I'd be happier at school if Wilma were in classes with me." She then refused to discuss the matter any further.

Seeing that the sessions were going nowhere, the psychiatrist asked her if she'd like to discontinue therapy. "Yes, if it is all right with you," was the reply. The man recorded that Helen was "borderline" in intelligence, citing her low scores on cognitive tests like the Stanford-Binet. He recommended that she discontinue school or have her academic program modified. "She is dull mentally, and she has a rigid mother who derives great satisfaction in having quadruplet daughters." It's safe to say this man would not have been amused to know the city was preparing to name Sadie Mother of the Year. Still, he doesn't appear to have once questioned her sanity or considered reporting her to authorities. Unlike the Louise Littles of the world, Sadie had the right to be a bad parent.

Sadie refused to accept the psychiatrist's recommendation regarding school, at least for the time being. She continued to observe Helen deteriorating, later telling NIMH researchers that Helen had begun to make sighing noises, snap her tongue, and "hatefully" comb her hair. She also became more destructive at home, breaking lightbulbs, kicking furniture, and running to her sisters' room to tear their clothing apart. She was more composed at school.

When Helen lost ten pounds from persistent vomiting, two family friends offered to take her in. The married couple believed they could save Helen if they gave her the right care. Teachers, too, thought Helen could thrive if only given permission. The quadruplets' homeroom teacher, one of the few to observe all four together, noted that it wasn't only Helen's mother but also her sisters who held her back. They'd always speak for her, instead of allowing her to express herself. Edna was particularly obnoxious—"so sure of herself" and always hogging the limelight. The teacher made a point to talk to Helen and ask her opinions about different matters. "She was just so tickled that somebody was noticing her," he later related. "She seemed starved for affection." Another teacher observed that, while Helen was clearly below average in brains, she was trying her best. Shouldn't that count for something?

Sadie would not permit her friends to take Helen, saying the quadruplets should be kept together. Even at this point in their lives, she was still very committed to equality among them. In fact she cared more about equality than excellence when it came to things like their grades. If the studious Edna achieved high marks, Sadie fretted she was getting too far ahead of the others. (So did Sarah, who worked frantically to keep up with her best friend.) Only a few months after declining the offer of a home for Helen, Sadie told school officials she was withdrawing her youngest, citing her poor academic performance. Helen's homeroom teacher protested that her potential was stifled and urged a provision for her to complete her final years. It would be such a shame for her to quit when she was so close to graduating. His objections were no use. Helen was disenrolled.

The sisters understood a different reason for her withdrawal than the one Sadie offered: Their parents were worried Helen would imperil their carefully cultivated image. In Sarah's words, "They felt that her masturbation made her so mentally retarded that her behavior would be a disgrace to them." They also worried the masturbation itself would be found out. By taking her out of school, they could dodge embarrassment at having "that kind of child" in public.

Shortly before Helen's withdrawal, there'd been an incident that exacerbated their fears. Helen had been staying after school, claiming to be studying in the library. One day Sadie went to check on her, finding her down the hall with her biology teacher. It was the former grade school janitor. He'd gone to college and gotten his teaching license. Helen denied any wrongdoing, but Sadie didn't believe her.

Edna, Sarah, and Wilma whispered their disapproval about Helen's dropping out. If they were being honest, they were nervous about what their peers would think. But it was primarily heartbreak for Helen that absorbed them. Wilma was the most despondent, begging to quit school and stay home with her sister.

When their shock wore off, the older sisters became emboldened. For the first time in her life, Edna refused to go along with Sadie and Carl's make-believe. Asked to pretend Helen had dropped out because of rheumatic fever, she relinquished her role as spokesperson. More and more, she began to stay home from school with abdominal or menstrual difficulties. Sarah, too, refused to uphold the pretense (though she happily stepped up as group representative). "I thought it was a big lie, and I was so annoyed," she later explained to the government researchers. Wilma, for her part, began to threaten her father whenever he knocked Helen around, dunked her head in a basin, or threatened even worse abuse. One day she looked him squarely in the eye and declared, "I'd like to do to you what you talk of and what you do to her and see how you'd feel."

But no one resisted more than Helen. The littlest sister "fought back like a tiger" whenever her father inflicted punishment. She'd kick and scream, and throw whatever she could at him. As Carl was often inebriated, she sometimes managed to overpower him. She took a more passive-aggressive approach with Sadie. If ever her mother tried to suggest she venture outside or run an errand, she'd slyly remind, "I'm supposed to be sick."

Of course Helen *was* sick, and severely so. She was having nightmares and walking in her sleep. She tossed so much in her cot that Sadie had to move her to a mattress on the floor. She also had tantrums and would slap herself, pull her hair, or strike out with her hands. Some experts alleged such behaviors were characteristic of early-stage schizophrenia, but her parents never suspected this or any other disorder to be underlying Helen's conduct. This might have been because diagnoses were not as important as they are today. Doctors didn't need to name a condition in order to treat and prescribe sedatives, often simply labeling people as anxious.

Furthermore, even if there were women like Little being held in asylums for paranoid tendencies, schizophrenia was presented to the public as a disease of docility and withdrawal. Popular magazines portrayed schizophrenics as white middle-class housewives who had something comparable to neurosis. This characterization stemmed from the psychoanalytic view of the condition, which stressed "reaction" to the pressures of modern life. (Swiss American psychiatrist Adolf Meyer used the word *reaction* in 1906 to describe temporary psychosis brought on by a deterioration of thinking habits under duress.) This perspective went even more mainstream the year Helen dropped out with the popular film *The Snake Pit*. Based on Mary Jane Ward's 1946 autobiographical novel of the same name, the drama portrayed a young woman who lost touch with reality, having to undergo therapy to resolve childhood hurt before she could regain her sanity. Only four years later, the widely referenced *Mental Disorders: Diagnostic and Statistical Manual*, now known as *DSM-I*, codified the notion that schizophrenia was a largely passive condition, resulting, at least in part, from early-life conflicts. The manual even used the word *reaction*.

Helen hardly resembled the withdrawn housewives of popular media. Moreover, for her parents to see the stirrings of madness in her would have required them to examine their parental failings. That was not something the Morloks were inclined to do.

Without her other half, Wilma had no choice but to try to join the other two at school. To be a full-fledged triplet, she had to improve her grades to Edna's and Sarah's levels. With diligence, she was able to score better, once even earning the highest grade in their typing class. According to their homeroom teacher, Sarah was delighted for her. Edna, on the other hand, had a look he'd never seen before. It was fleeting, but he was sure he wasn't mistaken: It was hate.

With Helen now out of the picture, Wilma became known as the amorous one. She would stand around her locker and meet boys, asking some of them to walk her home. She once startled her mother by announcing that she'd like to have intercourse. She claimed a girl at school had told her it was possible to do so without getting pregnant. Sadie assured her that wasn't true, so she shouldn't try. "I couldn't get pregnant if he just fingered me," Wilma retorted. Sadie replied that this would only work her up to have intercourse. No, said Wilma. She'd already been felt by one boy without it going any further.

Had she confessed this a few months before, Wilma might have endured brutal punishment, in addition to being dragged before the family psychiatrist. Now Sadie was too overwhelmed by caring for Helen to do much about Wilma's behavior. By late spring 1949, Helen was mostly catatonic. She would sit and stare into space for prolonged periods of time. She'd also wander around the house like a zombie. As her sisters' graduation approached in June, her crying spells increased.

These behaviors were more indicative of the schizophrenia that Carl and Sadie would have encountered in the popular press. Still, Sadie persisted in thinking Helen's deviance was to blame. She later claimed Helen was plagued by remorse for her ways, asking, "Mother, do you think that if I had not been quite so sex crazy I could have concentrated more and finished with the other girls?"

"I suppose so," Sadie recalled replying to that question, "and now I want to know just how much of what I am thinking is true."

Helen knew she meant wrongdoing with the janitor and admitted he had fondled her, both in grade and high school, Sadie would tell experts. In grade school, the fondling had occurred daily—sometimes up to four times a day—in a stairway. The man made her promise to keep it a secret from her mother. At the very least, she should keep quiet until she turned eighteen. Helen also told of other boys and male teachers touching her over the years. The boys were a group of three, who would take her to a room adjoining a laboratory. They would go in one at a time and have their turn with her.

Sadie replied that it was indeed her misdeeds that had prevented her from succeeding in school. The idea that her daughter had been victimized in these encounters didn't seem to cross her mind, perhaps because society adamantly denied that sexualized women could be raped. In many states, non-virgins had no legal case against their assailants, as they were thought to already be defiled. Nor did Black women, who were believed to be dirty by nature.

Hearing her mother's rebuke, Helen turned bitter. She claimed she would never have gone to school if she wasn't so wild about being pleasured.

Sadie considered this. "It's true that you missed less than the other girls," she said, referring to Helen's surprisingly stellar attendance.

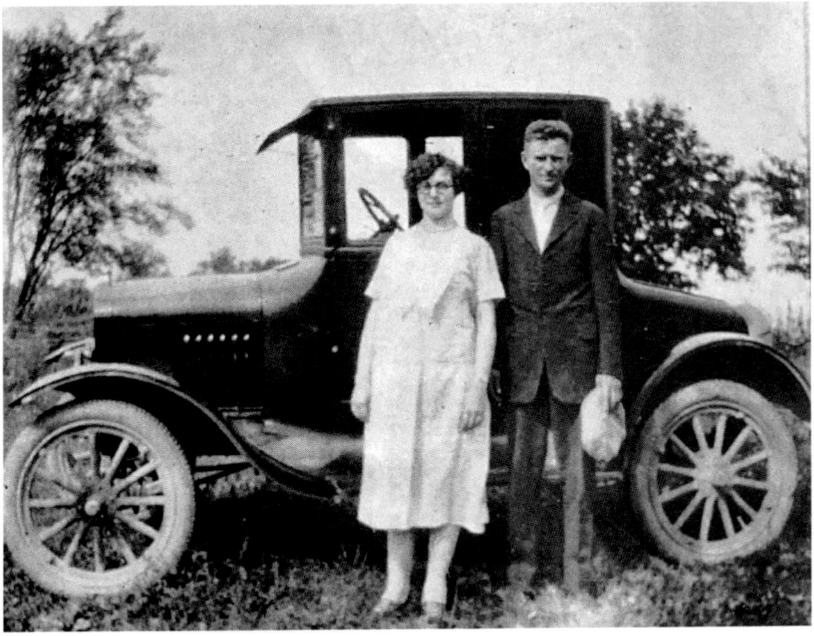

Sadie and Carl Morlok, undated. *(Sarah Morlok Cotton collection)*

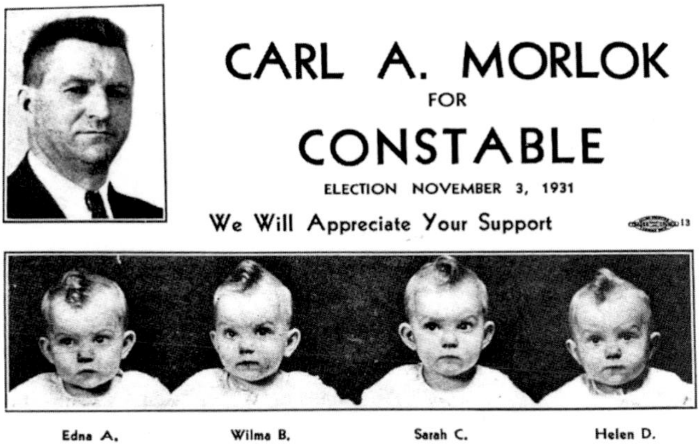

Carl Morlok's campaign card, 1931. *(Sarah Morlok Cotton collection)*

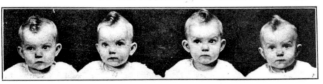

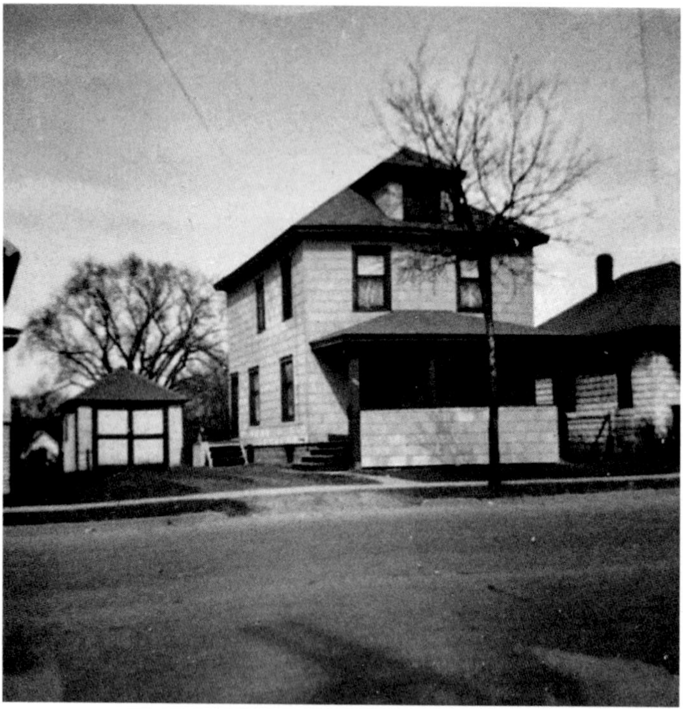

The Morlok family home at 1023 East Saginaw Street, 1957. *(Sarah Morlok Cotton collection)*

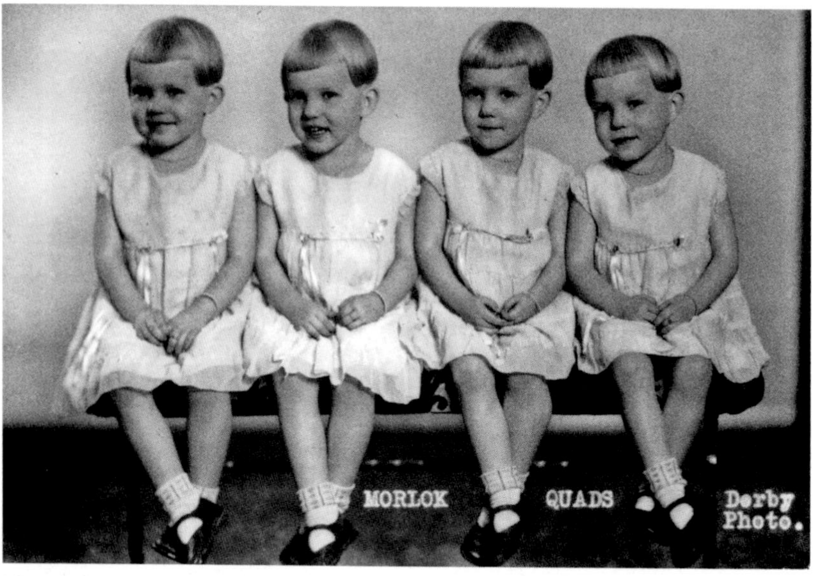

The quadruplets at three years old, taken by Derby Studio, 1933. *(Capital Area District Library collection)*

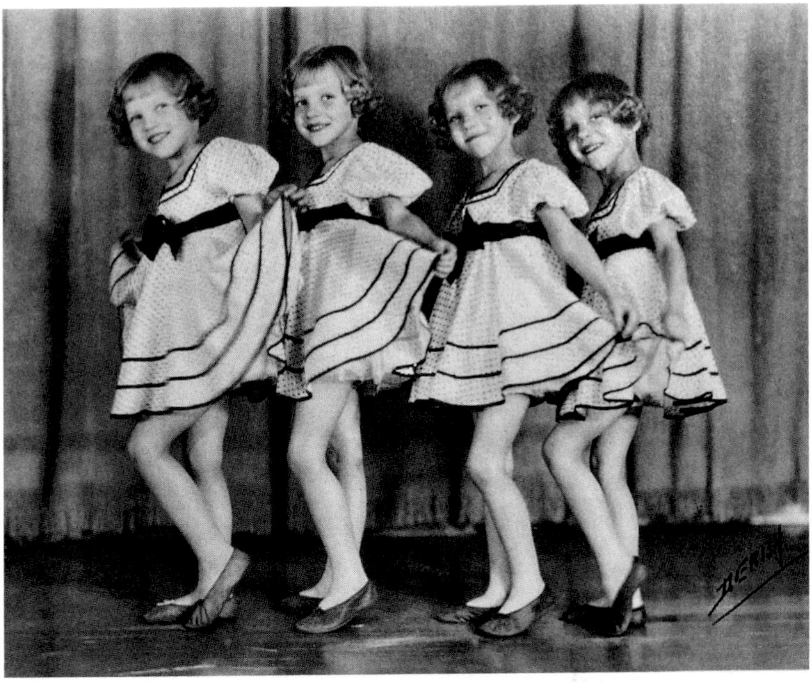

The quadruplets at five years old, taken by Derby Studio, 1935. *(Capital Area District Library collection)*

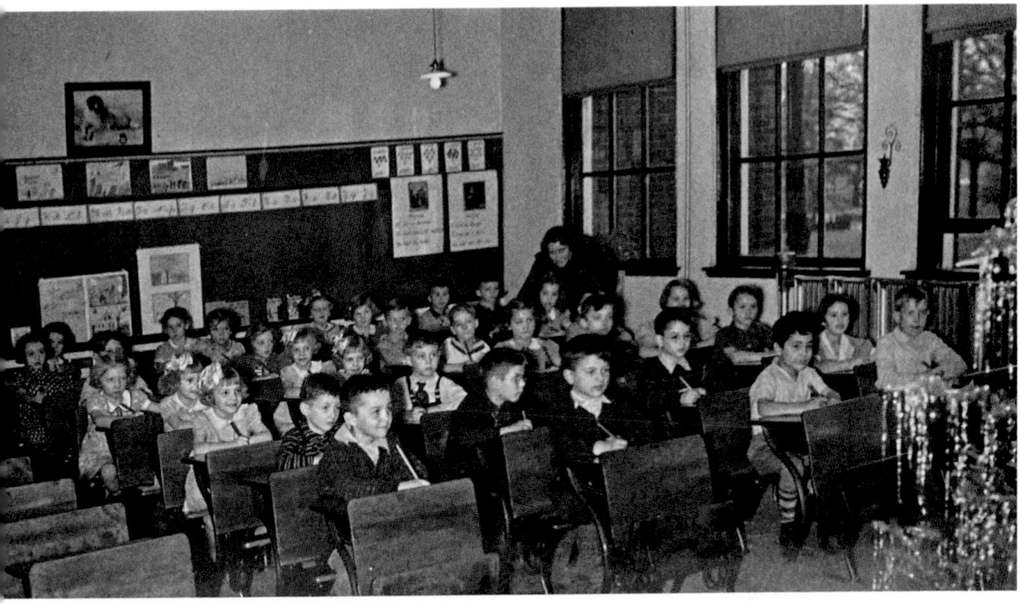

The quadruplets' first-grade class, undated. *(Sarah Morlok Cotton collection)*

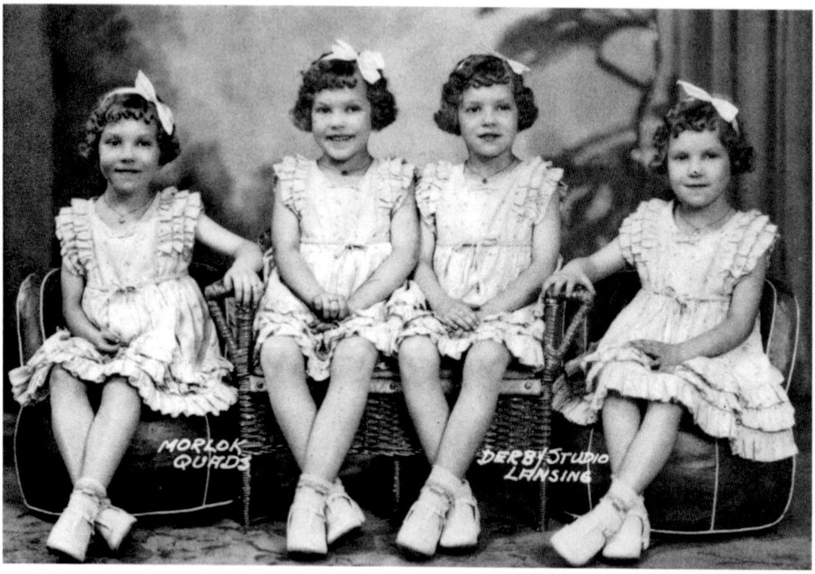

The quadruplets at seven years of age, taken by Derby Studio, 1937. *(Capital Area District Library collection)*

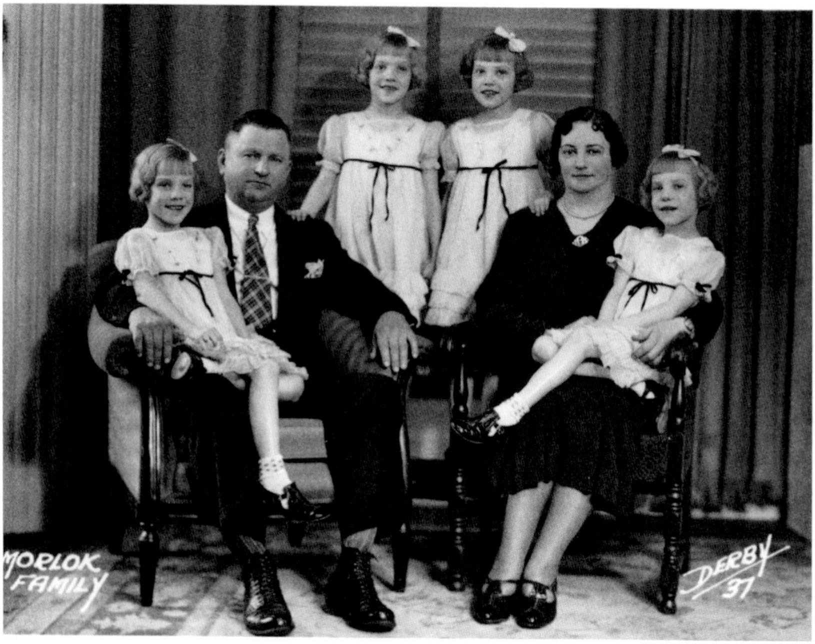

The Morlok family, taken by Derby Studio, 1937. *(Capital Area District Library collection)*

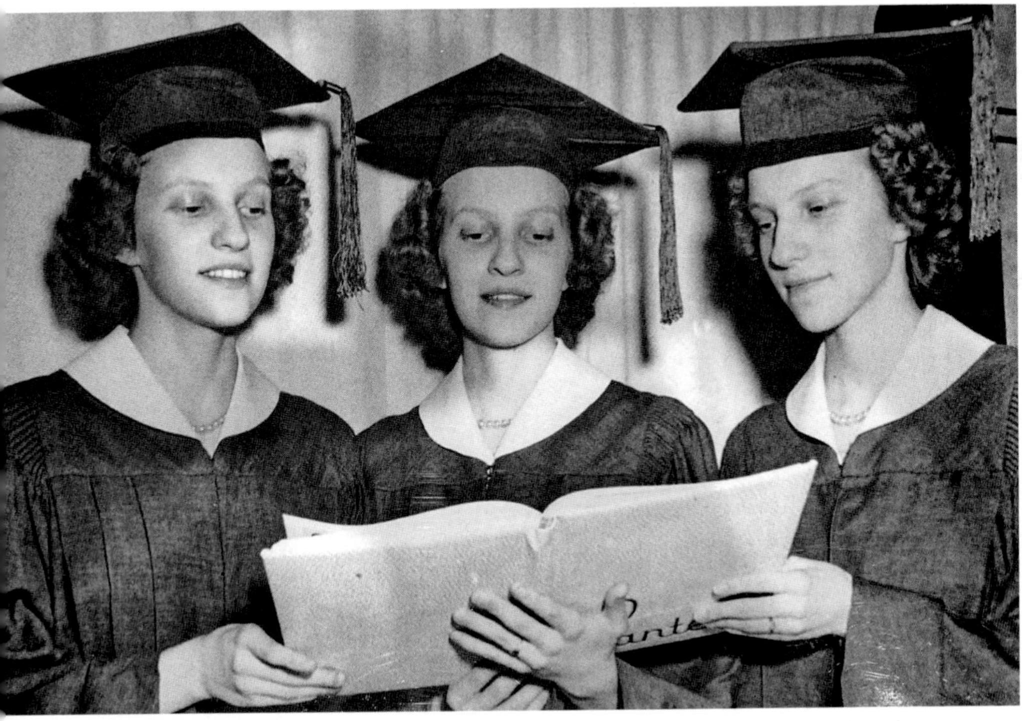

Edna, Sarah, and Wilma Morlok in their high school graduation gowns, 1949. *(Sarah Morlok Cotton collection)*

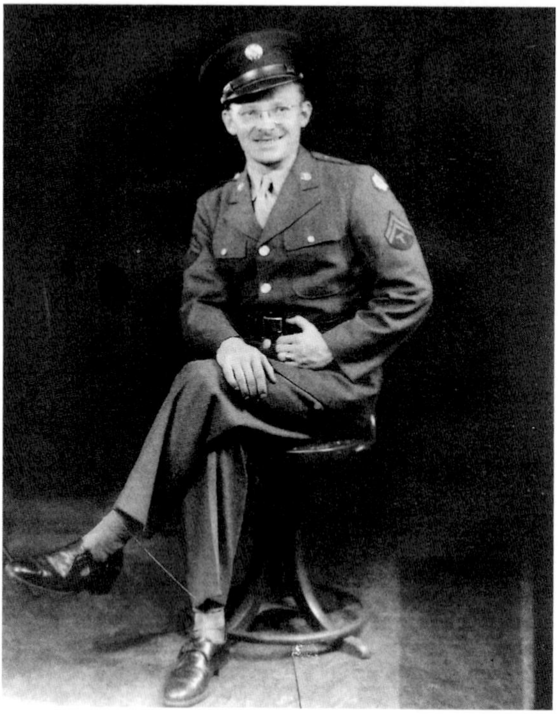

David Rosenthal in his military uniform, taken by his brother Arthur, undated. *(Ian Rosenthal collection)*

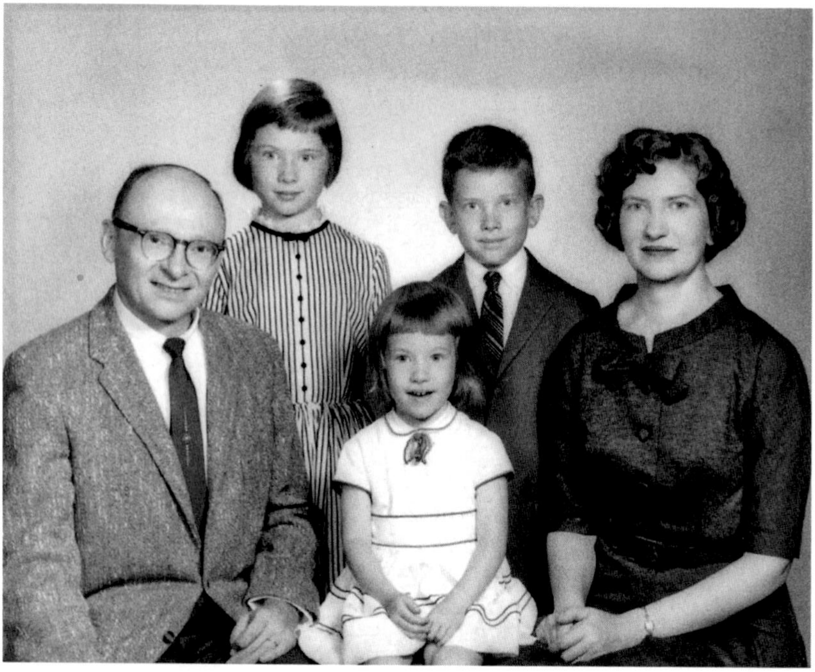

The Rosenthal family, in a 1961 photo taken by Arthur Rosenthal. Clockwise: David, Laura, Scott, Marcia, and Amy. *(Ian Rosenthal collection)*

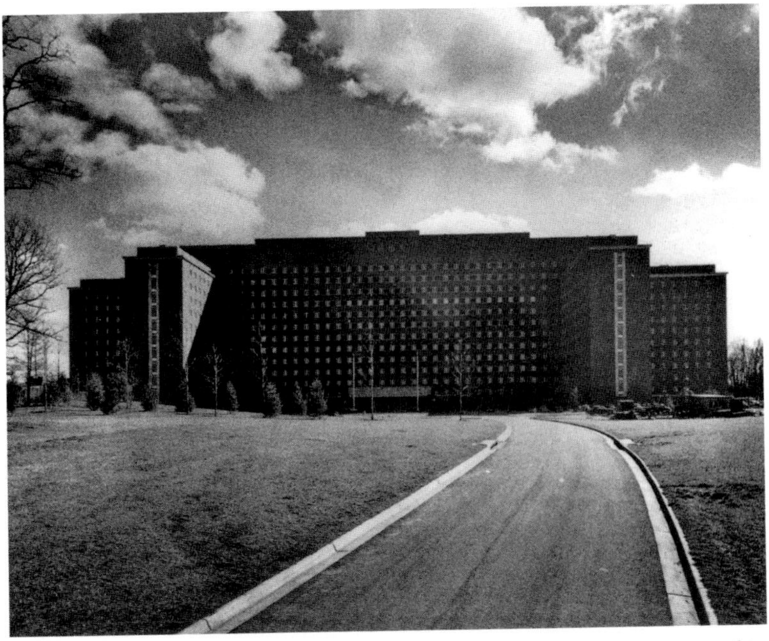

The NIH Clinical Center, also known as Building 10, around 1960. It opened in 1953 and was the tenth structure built on the Bethesda, Maryland, campus. *(NIH History Office)*

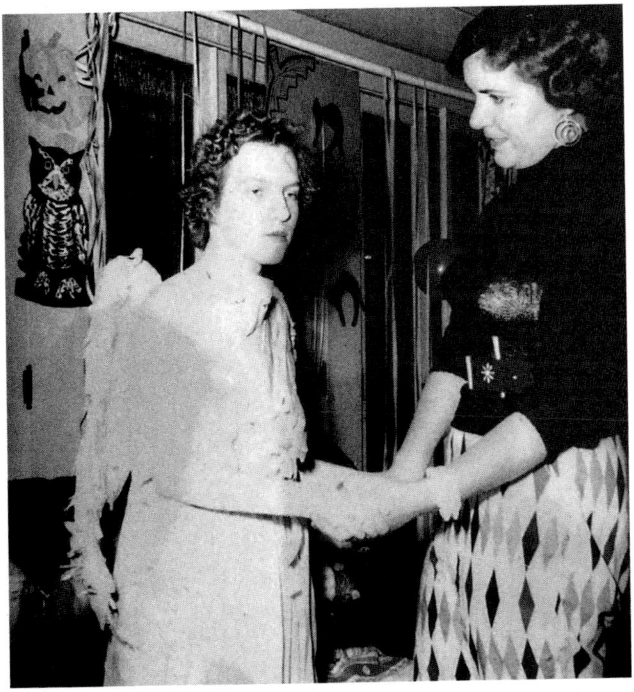

Helen Morlok with a nurse at a 1957 Halloween party at the NIH Clinical Center. *(Sarah Morlok Cotton collection)*

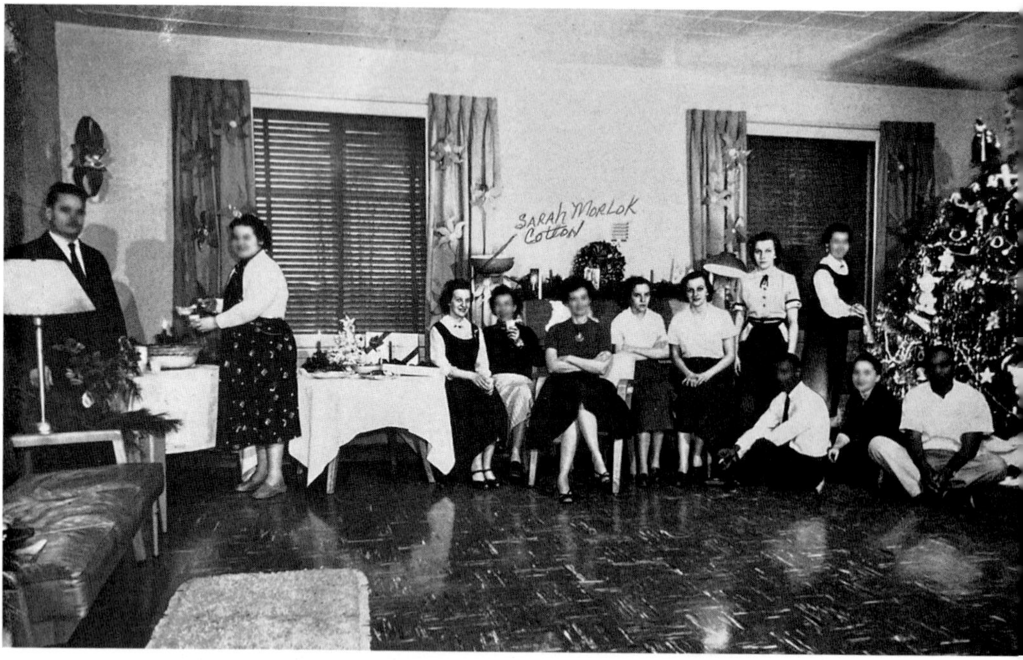

The Morlok quadruplets at a Christmas party at the NIH Clinical Center, undated. *(Sarah Morlok Cotton collection)*

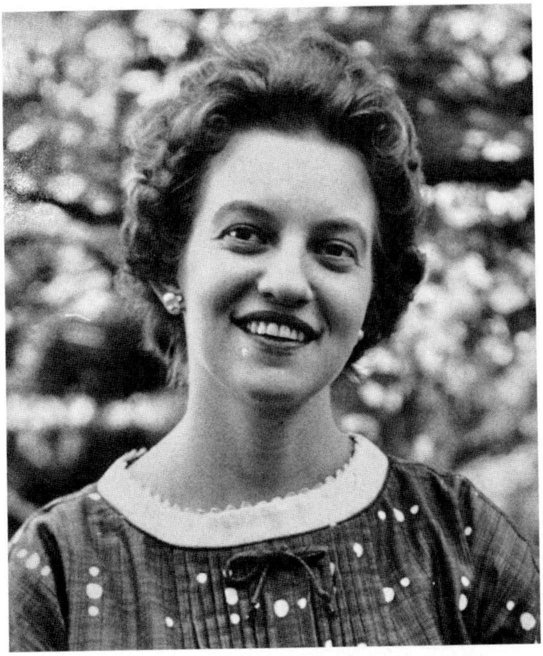

Sarah Morlok, outside the NIH Clinical Center, 1957. *(Sarah Morlok Cotton collection)*

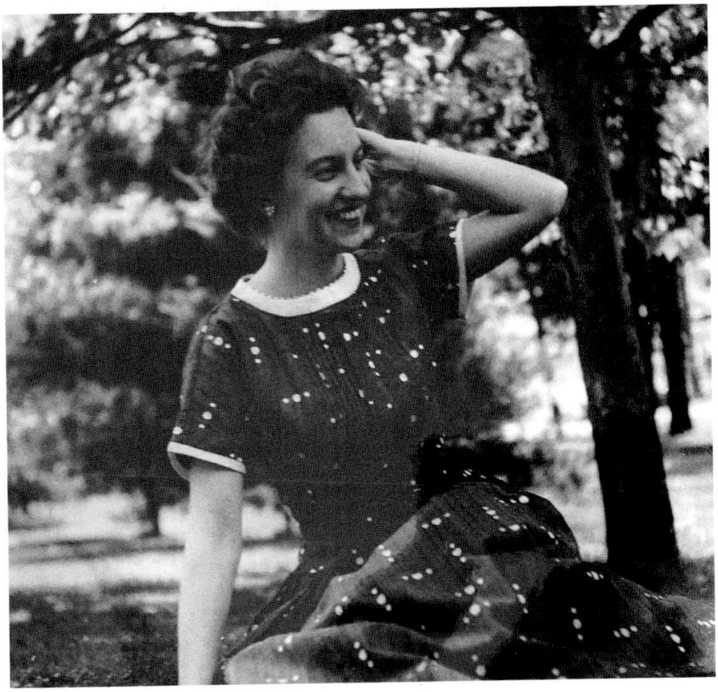

Sarah Morlok, on the lawn outside the NIH Clinical Center, 1957. *(Sarah Morlok Cotton collection)*

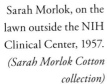

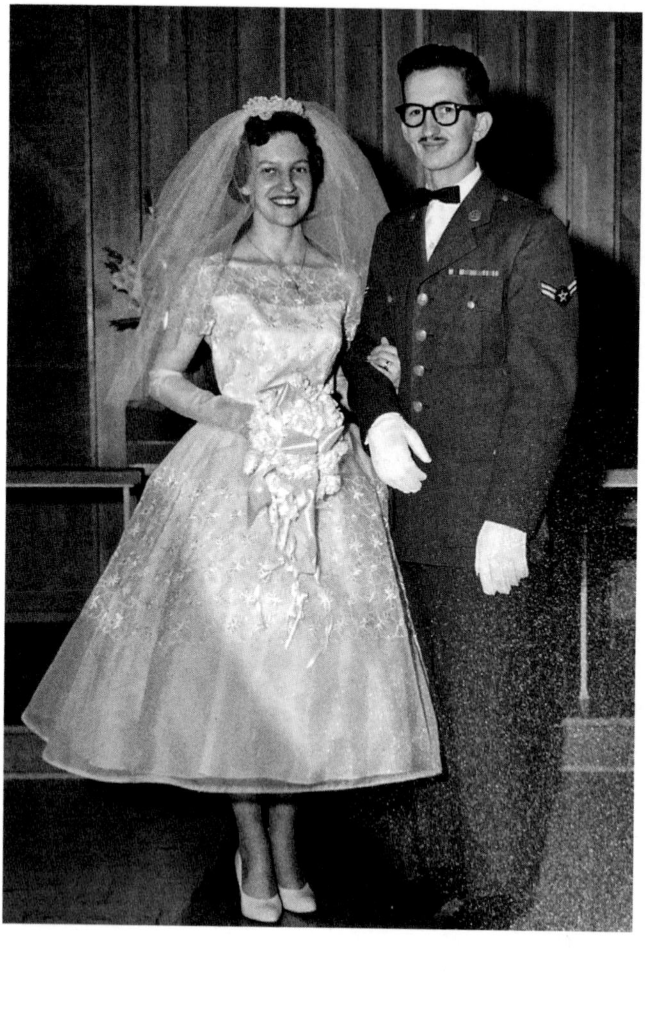

Sarah Morlok's wedding to George Cotton, 1961. *(Sarah Morlok Cotton collection)*

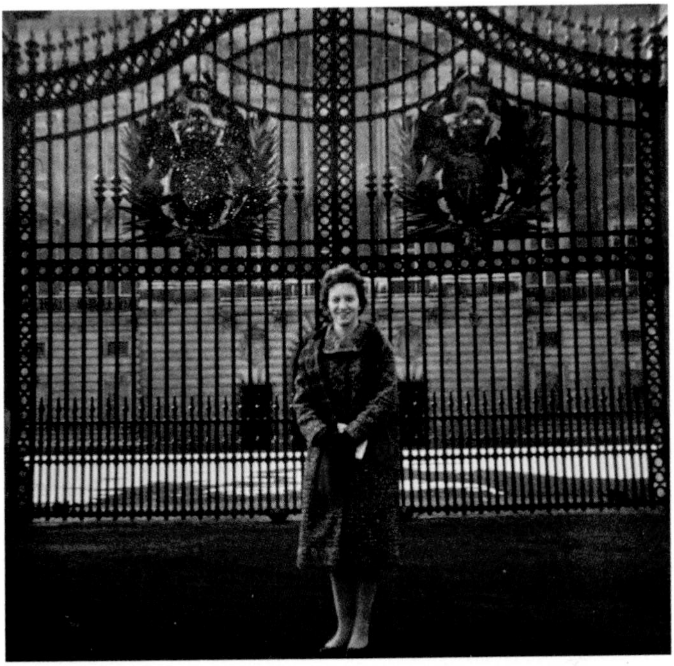

Sarah Cotton, standing at the gates of Buckingham Palace, undated. *(Sarah Morlok Cotton collection)*

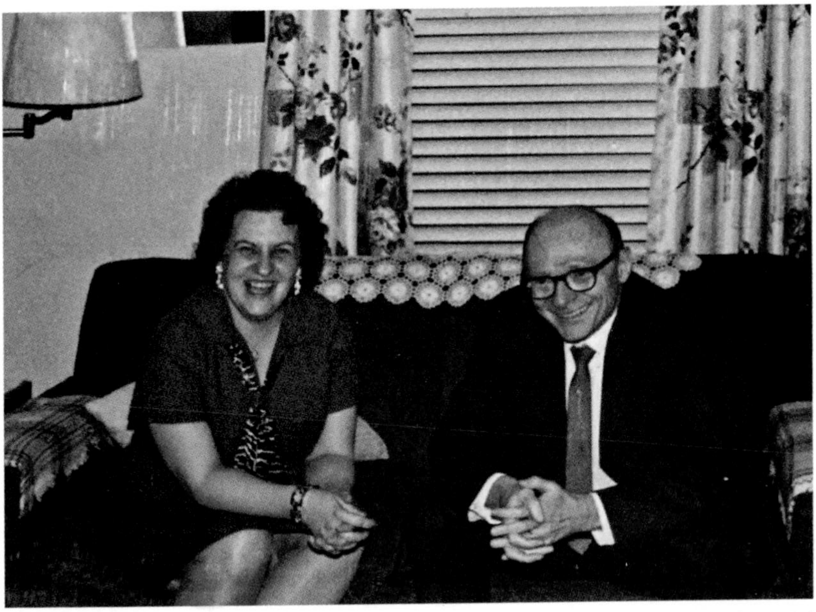

Edna Morlok and David Rosenthal at the Morlok family home, undated. *(Sarah Morlok Cotton collection)*

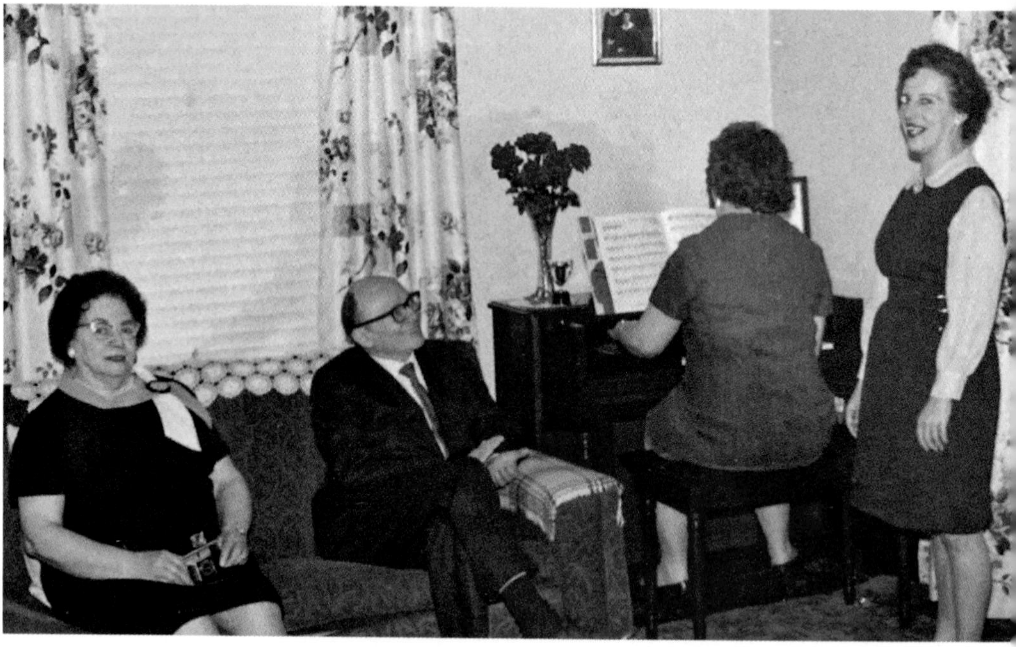

David Rosenthal visiting the Morlok family home in an undated photo. From left to right: Sadie Morlok, David Rosenthal, Edna Morlok, Helen Morlok. *(Sarah Morlok Cotton collection)*

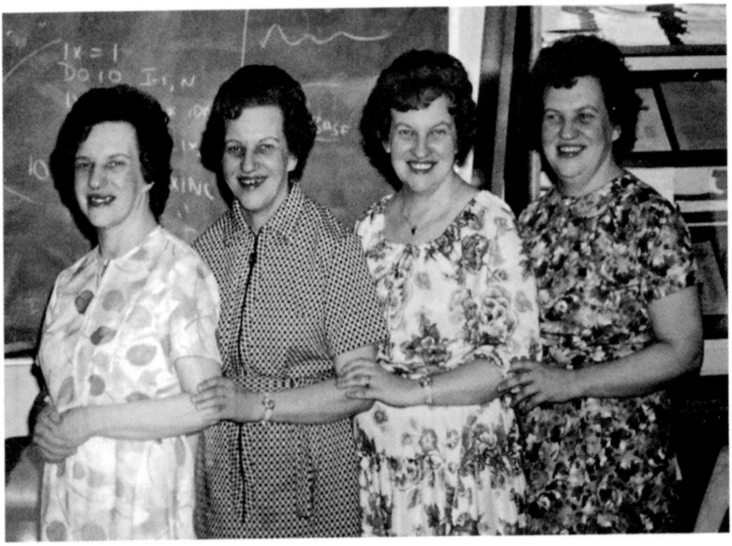

The Morlok sisters, undated. From left to right: Helen, Wilma, Sarah, and Edna. *(Sarah Morlok Cotton collection)*

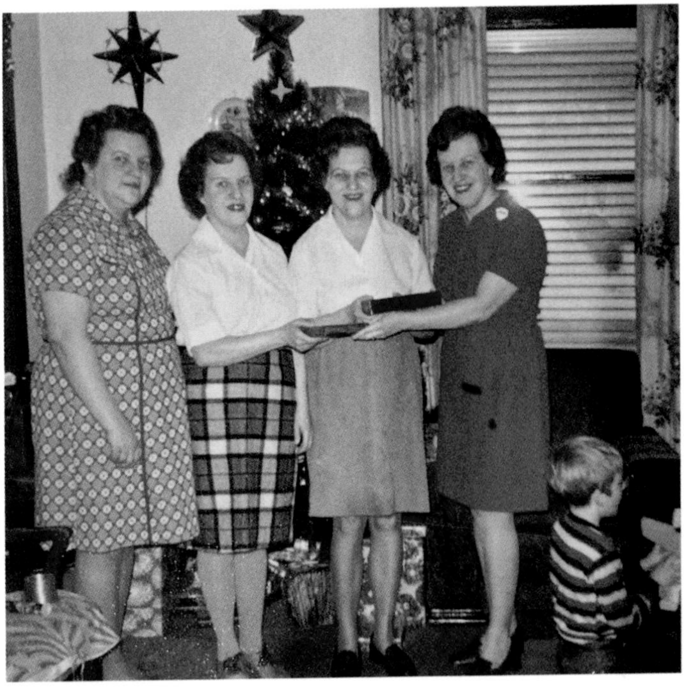

Christmas photograph of the Morlok sisters, undated. From left to right: Edna, Helen, Wilma, and Sarah. *(Sarah Morlok Cotton collection)*

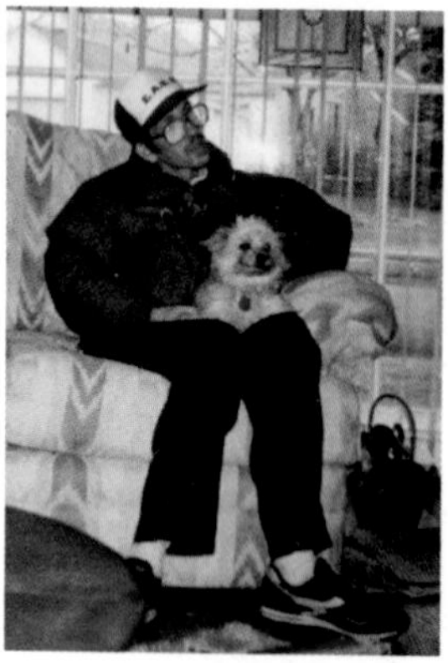

Bill Cotton, taken by his AIDS buddy Suellen Hozman, undated. *(Suellen Hozman collection)*

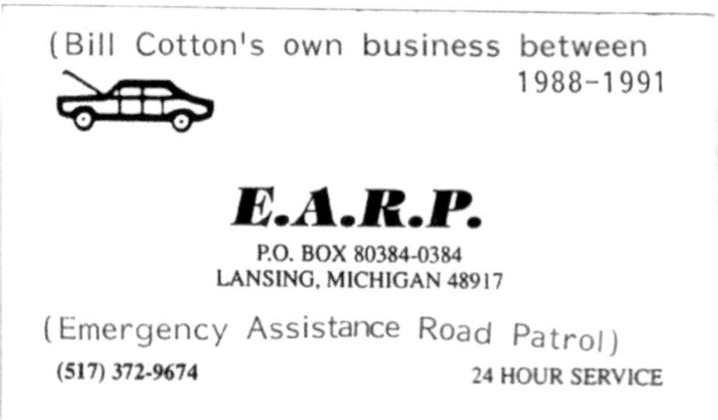

(Bill Cotton's own business between 1988–1991

E.A.R.P.

P.O. BOX 80384-0384
LANSING, MICHIGAN 48917

(Emergency Assistance Road Patrol)

(517) 372-9674 24 HOUR SERVICE

Bill Cotton's business card for his volunteer "Emergency Assistance Road Patrol," September 2022. *(Suellen Hozman collection)*

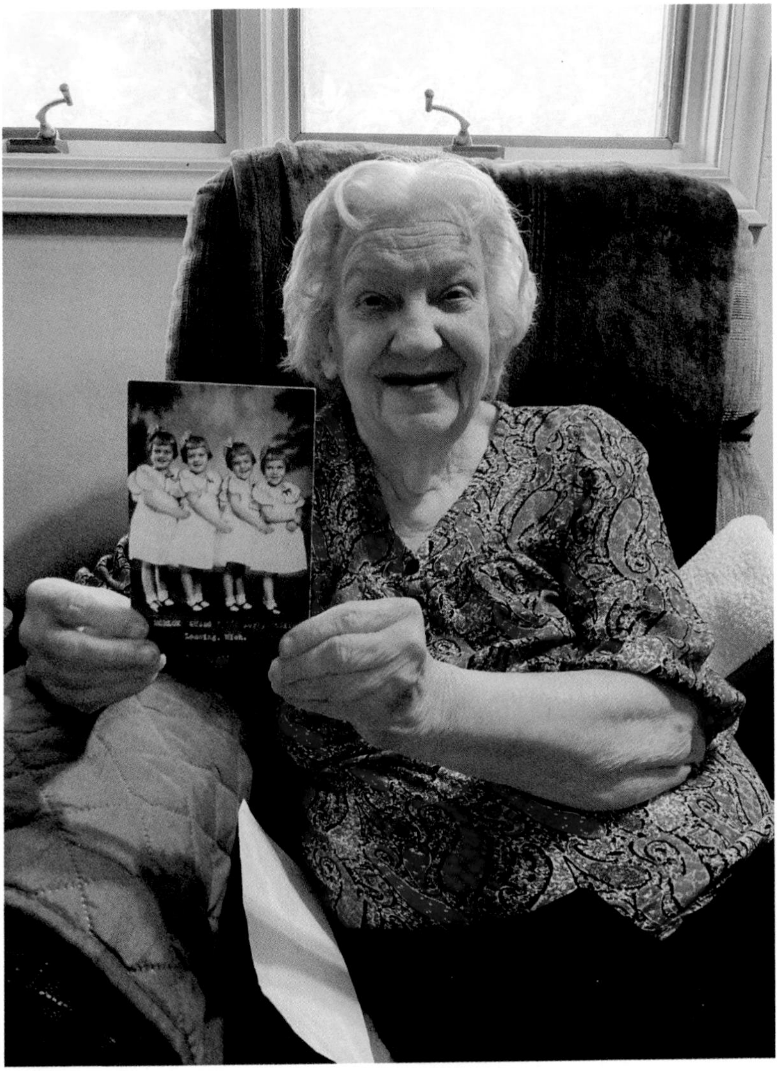

Sarah Cotton at age ninety-two, with a picture of the four sisters, May 2022. *(Author collection)*

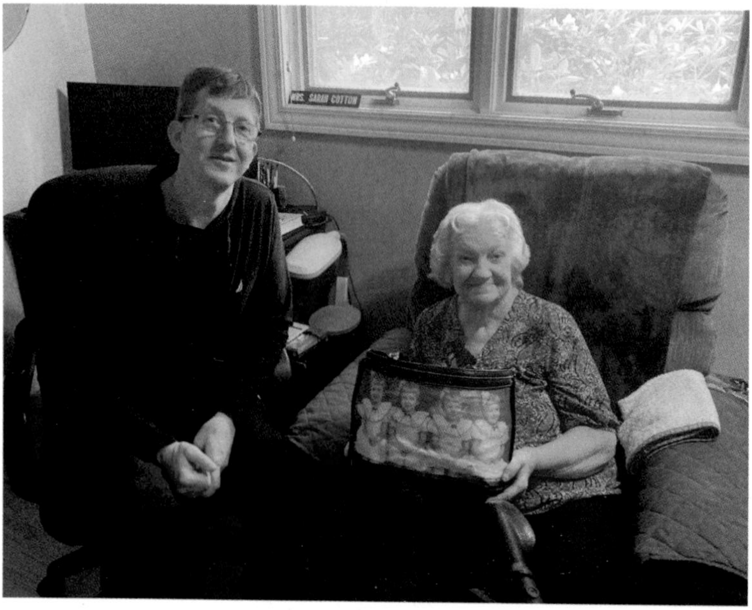

David and Sarah Cott
at her retirement home
May 2022. *(Author collection)*

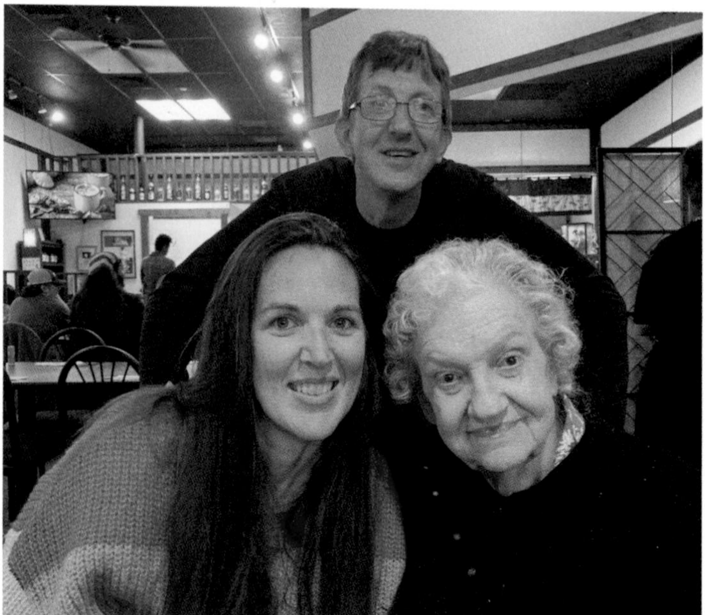

The author with David and Sarah Cotton, taken by Zaidi Yu, September 2022. *(Author collection)*

In the days leading up to her sisters' graduation, Helen let her contempt for her mother be known. Whenever her father would discuss his work schedule, which involved taking action against the "bad guys," she'd remark that her mother deserved the same treatment. She deeply resented Sadie for not allowing her to reach this milestone along with her sisters. It didn't help that Edna and Sarah were going to receive special recognition at the graduation ceremony for being in the National Honor Society. They were ranked 30th and 43rd in their class of 333, though the principal later told NIMH researchers their grades "were a reflection of their personality and terrific drive."

Carl was also struggling with his daughters' rite of passage. As the big day approached, he threatened he'd never survive the ceremony. He was desperate for them to forgo the event for his sake. Perhaps a father as tyrannical as Carl was bound to loathe the idea of their gaining the possibility of employment and independence. Perhaps, too, he was compelled by the sense that if society did not recognize his children as adults, he could continue to grope them.

Whatever its rationale, Carl's fantasy suffered a tremendous blow in June 1949, when Edna, Wilma, and Sarah received their diplomas. Despite his rancor, Carl did attend the ceremony. So did Helen, struggling to hold back her own emotions. At least for a moment, the two most antagonistic family members were united in sentiment. Both mourned the end of an era and braced for the one to come.

Chapter Seven

One by one, they'd come into the world, and in the very same order, they lost touch with it.

Edna surely never imagined it would go this way, especially after becoming the first to take an adult job. Shortly after her high school graduation, the eldest accepted a stenography position at a local government agency. Never had she felt so liberated. She made friends of her very own, going to the movies with them and receiving a deluge of Christmas cards that year. ("I'll catch up with you," said Sarah, after counting and finding she had fewer greetings from contacts at her own new place of employment.) Edna earned her own money and could afford new clothing and even home furniture. She volunteered to buy a living room set after the family had to get rid of a bedbug-ridden couch. She and Sarah had been quite embarrassed by the austere state of the room—there were only two rocking chairs.

Edna's bliss didn't last long, as her father and male co-workers quickly pushed her to a breaking point. Carl worked in the same building and insisted on accompanying her to and from the office, sometimes watching her work. He seldom said anything, just standing there and staring as she went through her tasks. He also demanded she come home with him for lunch. If she wasn't ready to leave when he wanted, he'd go out to his car and lay on the horn.

More troubling, though, were Carl's threats of serious illness. Edna shared a desk and telephone with two people who'd recently been discharged from a tuberculosis sanitarium. When her father found this out, he began to warn that she'd catch the dreaded disease. Edna began to compulsively sanitize the telephone with alcohol. That fall, she caught a cold and cough, which Carl assured her were the beginning symptoms of tuberculosis. She went for a chest X-ray and was cleared. Perhaps, said Carl, the illness was simply not advanced enough to show up on the scan and the doctor was only telling her it was negative to protect her from worrying. Fear for her health made Edna extremely timid on the job, and her employers took note. To them, she appeared stand-offish, hesitating to take papers from colleagues and leaning away from conversation. How were they to know that she was deeply afraid of contagion and of anyone who might be a vector of it? That she was being manipulated by a man who was absolutely obsessed with protecting the borders of his daughters' bodies, lest anything dangerous enter?

At twenty, Edna began to have crying spells. Carl assured her she was working herself to death. He also continued to threaten that *he* was dying, as this still got a rise out of her.

Then one day Carl's fears of perilous penetration were nearly realized. An elevator operator attempted to rape Edna. While the two of them were alone in the contraption, he stopped it between floors and pushed her against the wall, taking his pants down and pressing himself against her. Edna kicked and screamed, somehow managing to get away and running for the nearby mayor's office. It was actually Carl whom she first came upon. "Oh, that fellow is all right," said her father, after hearing what had happened. "He wouldn't do anything. Maybe he was just intoxicated and scared you." Seeing Edna was not satisfied with this, he added that "these things happen" from time to time, so she might as well get used to it.

After all his supposed preparing his daughters for sexual assault and his talk about the dangers of the workplace, he claimed not to believe it when rape was attempted. It's possible he didn't think Edna to be credible in her current psychological state. It's also possible he did believe her but felt too ineffectual to do anything. His impotence had become so severe that he now hadn't had sex with his wife in years. He was not only embarrassed about this but also obsessed with the virility he perceived in others, often accusing Sadie of being attracted to younger, fitter men. But it really seems that Carl imagined very particular villains, whom this man simply did not resemble. When people in his circles violated women, it didn't count.

Soon after the assault, Edna began to complain of aching in her shoulder and chest. A doctor found she had low iron in her blood, prescribing vitamin shots and iron tablets. Then, while attending a funeral, she experienced what some would call her first hallucination. She saw her father in the casket. The image haunted her for the next month, during which time she became further run-down. "I wish I had never gone to that funeral," she told her mother. "I haven't felt well since." By Christmas, she had awful sinus problems. Come the new year, her ailments expanded to include insomnia and stomach spasms. All this time, Carl went on about her having tuberculosis.

Edna claimed to be distraught by the vision of her dead father, and she probably was, having long been close to him. But was there also something wishful about what she conjured? Did the idea of losing Carl bring as much comfort as it did distress?

In April 1951, the eldest quadruplet took a leave of absence from work. Co-workers called the house to express concern, but Sadie didn't permit any of them to speak with her. In June, Edna officially resigned. She now complained that her neck bones were slipping out of place. She perched on her knees and elbows till they bled, and walked and talked in her sleep. "I don't know where it is," she'd say, pacing back and forth. "I can't find it." Sarah was so troubled by the sight and sound of her that Sadie moved Edna to another room.

Fearing Edna's condition would reflect poorly on the Morlok brand, Carl began to threaten murder-suicide. "I'll stop it all if there is any question of mental trouble in this family," he told Edna. "I'm physically ill. You're mentally ill. I have guns and I may use them, and I'll not leave your mother out." She had no reason not to believe him, no reason to think he wouldn't actually sacrifice his own flesh and blood to save face.

With Sadie busy cooking, running errands, and seeing that they didn't run up the gas or water bills (which incensed Carl), Helen stepped up to care for her sister. She waited on Edna and served her meals in bed. In the time since the high school graduation, the youngest sister had done relatively well. Though she'd initially resented having to launder and iron her sisters' nice work clothes, and though she was forced to do all of the dirty work from taking out the garbage to emptying Carl's odorous spittoon, she had adjusted well to home life. This probably had much to do with the facts that she was no longer being compared with her sisters and her father was growing too invalid to keep up his torments. Carl still insulted her and went out of his way to step on her feet when he crossed the room, but he simply didn't have it in him to push her around like before. All the same, it was surely a sign of calamity that the most troubled sister was now holding things together.

In September, Edna recovered enough to help Helen with some of the housework, and in November, she returned to work. A few months later, she became extremely paranoid that people were looking at her and threatened to take her own life. Her doctor referred her to Mercywood Sanitarium in Ann Arbor. Ever the cheapskate, Carl wanted a public asylum for his daughter. However, great stigma surrounded these institutions—they were for perceived cretins and hopeless cases—and so he was persuaded to pony up some money for the private Mercywood, which was staffed by nuns. Sarah and one of Sadie's brothers also contributed to Edna's hospital costs.

There she was diagnosed with acute schizophrenia, undifferentiated subtype, a no-longer-recognized subtype for cases in which someone did not meet the criteria for a singular type, such as paranoid, catatonic, or hebephrenic. (Paranoid type denoted someone who appeared to be primarily affected by suspicious thinking or behavior; catatonic type denoted someone who appeared to mainly suffer from immobility or lack of communication; and hebephrenic type denoted a person characterized by incoherent or bizarre thoughts and behaviors.) The psychiatrist there, Dr. Leonard Himler, cited Edna's experience at the funeral as her first psychotic manifestation, also recording that she was prone to paranoia, insomnia, vomiting, moaning, groaning, trembling, chewing her fingers, and running her hands through her hair.

Carl and Sadie provided background information about Edna, playing down their overbearing ways. They claimed, for instance, that Edna was uninterested in dating, rather than that she was forbidden from it, and they made no mention of the enormous pressure upon the quadruplets to uphold a certain image. In all fairness, they probably didn't grasp the psychic demands of constantly being in the public eye. When privately talking with professionals, however, Sadie conveyed some misgivings about Carl's mental state. She said he often tried to slap her and that he was irritable, profane, and fault-finding. He heard noises when no one else did, shouted, paced, and sulked for days if food was not made just so.

When Dr. Himler questioned Carl about these behaviors, Carl was furious. He asked Sadie how the man had come by the information. Sadie suggested it was the family doctor. She then had to call her scapegoat in tears to tell him not to leave his office, as Carl was outside in the parking lot with a gun. Somehow nothing tragic happened, but thereafter, Carl suspected his wife of turning on him. Whenever she met privately with Dr. Himler, he'd stand right outside the door.

Edna endured a round of convulsant electroshock for her ailments, but because she suffered from respiratory difficulties, clinicians were reluctant to repeat such a forceful therapy. They switched her to a form of electroshock that did not produce convulsions and Metrazol, a drug injected to induce seizures, which were believed to alleviate psychosis. Patients compared Metrazol therapy to such sensations as being roasted alive and having the skull bones spliced open; and in 1939, the New York State Psychiatric Institute had found that 43 percent of patients suffered spinal fractures from the treatment. But the Hungarian physician who'd pioneered the treatment insisted "nothing less than a shock to the organism [was] powerful enough to break the chain of noxious processes that leads to schizophrenia." The same rationale was offered for electroshock. "The greater the damage [to the brain], the more likely the remission of psychotic symptoms," wrote Georgetown and George Washington University researcher Walter Freeman, who is best remembered for performing Rosemary Kennedy's botched lobotomy in 1941.

After five of these combined treatments, Edna's panic and anxiety did ease, and she claimed to have no more delusions. Though still aloof and withdrawn, she was discharged. Once at home, her condition worsened. She complained of headaches, nausea, inability to think, and vision trouble. She also had the sensation of something opening and closing in her head. "Oh, dear," she began to repeat.

Edna's sisters were distraught about her hospitalization. Wilma was even beginning to show signs of her own breakdown. Claiming worry about her elder sibling, she began to vomit at her new secretarial job. It had taken her longer to gain employment, as she could not type or take shorthand as well as the others, and then she'd been let go from her first two jobs. After one of these dismissals, her father had gone in and threatened her boss that his friends in the government would take action if he didn't hire Wilma back. The man replied that he didn't work in the public sector and so he couldn't be intimidated. Carl was surely livid to be spoken to this way, but he didn't press the matter.

Wilma was growing terrified of one of her present employers, who once said to her, "I sure do like women." She couldn't concentrate and, according to a co-worker, would "ruin an afternoon and just be dazed and sort of sit and putter and not quite know where to start or what to do." Another of her bosses wanted to fire her, but he was afraid she'd do something desperate if he did.

Sadie wondered if she should take Edna and Wilma away, perhaps to see family. She had not been close to her siblings in years but felt a visit might be good for the two. Carl accused her of plotting to make floozies of them, saying, "You just want to get them started running around." Sarah also didn't want them to go, scared about being left alone with her father. Ever since Edna had become incapacitated, he'd redirected his affection toward her. She considered moving out of the house and renting a room at the YWCA, but was too afraid Carl would take his rage at her abandonment out on the others. He'd recently kicked a frying pan into Helen's face, chipping her front tooth and cutting the roof of her mouth.

It's unclear if tongues were beginning to wag beyond the quadruplets' work circles. During these tumultuous times, no one outside the family ever spoke to them about mental illness, although an elder Sarah would relate her belief that people *did* know, they were just too polite to broach the subject.

As time went on, Wilma's condition at work worsened. She would throw up as soon as she finished eating and then not even move to clean it up. She began to take her lunch in the restroom, prompting other women to sneer and call her names. It didn't help when Carl began to haunt her and Sarah at their jobs, nor when a worker in the building tried to force himself on her. This man cornered her in the washroom, pulled up her dress, yanked down her panties, and exposed himself. She screamed and ran to tell her supervisor, who informed her that her assailant was a very important man and so there wasn't much to be done.

After this essential life lesson that powerful men had carte blanche rights to assault, Wilma began to tell Sarah that men in the office were bothering her. She said they were trying to make her do things that she didn't want to do. She sometimes passed the night just sitting in a chair, as if keeping guard. One day she came home from work in shambles. She was crying, pacing, and rubbing her hands together. After dinner, she went to the living room and tried to bury her head in the newspaper, but couldn't bring herself to read. When Carl got up to adjust the radio, she ran to her room sobbing. Sadie followed after her, asking what was wrong. Wilma couldn't answer and just stared at the wall. Thinking she wanted to be alone, Sadie turned to go. "Someone is bothering me," she exclaimed. "I am pinned down. I am bothered by someone, and they want to fight, and I don't want to fight. Them people are just fighting." She wondered if the reverend at their church could preach a sermon to make people leave her alone.

When Edna heard Wilma upstairs, she began to grow hysterical herself. She, too, feared someone was after her. Sadie managed to calm them both down, giving Wilma sedatives to get her through the night. The next day, Wilma drooled at all of her meals and was unable to swallow. She insisted that someone was telling her to keep her head down and not look around. She now identified one of the voices as belonging to the vice president of her company, who'd once faulted her for a mistake.

It certainly seems that Wilma's hallucinations, like Edna's, were fueled by real events. But even when she sought care, no medical expert made a connection. Literature on schizophrenia had largely failed to capture the role of traumatic events—sexual or otherwise—in the development of psychosis, postulating some intrinsic origin or an external stressor like family conflict. In his much-revered 1911 treatise *Dementia Praecox, or the Group of Schizophrenias*, which had renamed dementia praecox as schizophrenia, Eugen Bleuler marveled that affected individuals experienced symbolic hallucinations as real bodily sensations: "Male patients have their semen drawn off; painful erections are stimulated . . . The women patients are raped and injured in the most devilish ways . . ." It didn't seem to cross Bleuler's mind that such hallucinations might be memories of actual experiences, not mere symbols of psychic conflicts. Bleuler's colleague Sigmund Freud was even more convinced that nothing in the world was ever as it appeared to be. So suspicious was Freud of secret meanings that he assigned taboo urges to individuals he'd never even met. After reading Daniel Paul Schreber's 1903 *Memoirs of My Nervous Illness*, in which the author revealed paranoid delusions suggestive of abuse suffered at the hands of his father, Moritz, the famed inventor of "purifying" orthopedic devices, Freud chalked the author's issues up to an Oedipal complex.

It wasn't just schizophrenia scholars who largely ignored trauma. The field of medicine, more broadly, was known for papering over violence. Perhaps the most egregious example: American clinicians had largely ignored questions of how slavery might devastate the psyche, some even asking how *emancipation* harmed the mental health of Black Americans. Nineteenth-century physician Samuel A. Cartwright invented the diagnosis of "drapetomania" to describe the desire to run away from one's master—so deluded was he about the pleasant nature of life in bondage. Cartwright also pointed toward the incidence of mental illness among free "Negroes" as proof that those of African descent didn't have the sophistication of mind or spirit to be unsupervised. There were probably more of his fingerprints than Bleuler's or Freud's on the case records of Louise Little, whose confinement at Kalamazoo State Hospital had now surpassed a decade. Doctors continued to describe her as "disagreeable and resistant," even forbidding visits from her minor children.

The midcentury saw renewed efforts to obscure the fact of rampant racial violence. When asylums began to promote intensive psychotherapy for all manner of mental illnesses—even schizophrenia—they did not usually offer this treatment to Black patients on the basis that they were too lacking in intellect to benefit from it. In lieu of hearing, among other troubles, of the all-too-real persecution of people living under Jim Crow, many asylum doctors simply labeled Black patients as maladjusted. Hospitalization thus tended to be iatrogenic, causing, rather than curing, mental trouble. Such was the case for Little, as one of her adult sons discovered upon visiting her in 1952. "She stared at me. She didn't know who I was. Her mind, when I tried to talk... was somewhere else."

White society continued to suppress the fact of ubiquitous violence against children, as well. Around the time that Wilma started to unravel, medical doctors were actually beginning to accept that physical abuse accounted for incidences of unexplained injuries in kids. (After thoroughly searching, they found no diseases to explain all the broken bones.) But according to cultural critic Richard Beck, they responded by using such tactful terms as *parental carelessness* and encouraging peers not to ask too many questions so as not to offend parents. This surely spoke "volumes about the [white] nuclear family's status in postwar society: the prestige, the respect, and especially the extraordinary degree of privacy that families regarded as their natural right." The idea that sexual abuse also pervaded respectable American homes remained even more unspeakable. Throughout the 1950s, society continued to present sexual abuse as anomalous—the kind of crime only sexual degenerates and people of color committed. This was true even though sex researcher Alfred Kinsey's extensive studies revealed incest and other intimate child sexual abuse to be extremely common.

Kinsey's findings on masturbation, homosexuality, and extramarital sex garnered great attention after their publication in 1953. By contrast, his discovery that grown men—but not grown women—frequently took sexual liberties with children barely registered in the public consciousness. According to Judith Herman, author of the 1981 book *Father-Daughter Incest*, Kinsey himself downplayed his findings, particularly regarding the fright and distress that 80 percent of women sexually abused as children reported they'd experienced immediately following the events. He "cavalierly belittled" such women and the prudish society he believed responsible for their trauma, writing, "It is difficult to understand why a child, except for cultural conditioning, should be disturbed at having its genitalia touched... Some of the more experienced students of juvenile problems have come to believe that the emotional reactions of the parents, police officers, and other adults who discover that the child has had such a contact, may disturb the child more seriously than the sexual contacts themselves."

Precisely because midcentury doctors and psychiatrists avoided reckoning with the realities of incest, the most common form of child sexual abuse, few had any sense of how—or even *that*—sexual abuse psychologically impacted victims. Which would explain why, when Wilma was admitted to the hospital in March 1953, psychiatrists didn't probe about her attacks, instead focusing on work stress and diagnosing her, just like her sister before her, with acute schizophrenia, undifferentiated type. Wilma stayed for more than a month, during which time a psychiatrist noted that she was very dependent, hanging on his arm. She underwent sixteen rounds of electroshock therapy, which she claimed freed her of delusions. But as with Edna, she worsened soon upon returning home.

Unbeknownst to the Morloks, a French surgeon had accidentally found a simple treatment for psychosis, which was now available in various European countries. In 1949, Henri Laborit had administered an antihistamine to soldiers going into surgery at a French military hospital in Tunisia. As the allergy drug was known to suppress the autonomic nervous systems, he thought giving it in a cocktail with other drugs would decrease the risk of surgical shock. Much to his surprise, the concoction, injected intravenously, transformed his patients' personalities, rendering them calm and relaxed. Once back in France, he arranged for a chemist at the antihistamine's manufacturing company to synthesize it, then for a few psychiatrists to administer the new compound—named chlorpromazine—to a patient of theirs. This man improved, and then another psychiatrist, Pierre Deniker, conducted clinical experiments, which found that many psychotics improved after being put on a regimen. Seventy-five milligrams seemed to do the trick. In 1952, the US pharmaceutical company Smith, Kline & French purchased rights for the drug and arranged for clinical testing on psychotic individuals at medical schools and private hospitals.

If Carl had known about the research under way, he might have tried to enroll his daughters in one of the trials in exchange for free treatment. He was perturbed when Wilma had relapsed after a costly private hospital stay. "We spent so much money on you, what are we going to do with you now?" he demanded to know. He spoke as if he didn't owe his livelihood to them.

"You don't know what to do with me, but Mother will know," Wilma replied.

It was true that Sadie had become more of an advocate. Edna's diagnosis seemed to have softened her. After years of blaming two of her daughters' behaviors on character flaws, she was beginning to understand that they were deeply troubled, likely because of the goings-on at home. Still, she largely blamed Carl, unable or perhaps unwilling to come to terms with her own role in their distress.

Sadie now scolded Carl for being so hard on the quadruplets and copping feels when he kissed them good night. (He deflected, saying her mind was in the gutter.) She also berated him for throwing himself a pity party when the family was in crisis. She was referring to the fact that Carl passed most days in the garage, drinking beer, insulting random people who walked by, and shooting animals who wandered into his yard. He was often overheard saying there were so many children growing up to be "rats in the city" that a person had to carry a gun. Then he'd fire a shot at some poor creature, a seeming stand-in for the human beings he loathed. Carl also now had a strange habit of shoveling too much coal in the furnace, then opening all the windows for the house to cool off. Once he passed out after a night of boozing, and Sadie decided to wrap him in bedsheets, then sew him in with a fishhook. He was incensed the following morning, trying to thrash his way to freedom. Sadie gently explained that the girls were very sick and it was time to shape up. If he didn't, she would do something drastic. What exactly, she didn't say.

Wilma was also reaching her limit with Carl. Once when he was going on about something, she got his gun and pointed it at him. Sadie was able to secure it from her before things turned deadly. Soon after this, Wilma returned to the hospital, claiming she wanted to drown herself in the river. During her stay, she asked her mother, "Was Dr. Haynes right?" She was referring to her childhood physician's remark that she was an institution case. Sadie's reply was never documented, but it's not unthinkable she now found it within herself to reassure Wilma what was happening was not her fault.

Following her second stay, a psychiatrist noted that Wilma, like her sister, had a strange habit of ignoring problems "by just smiling in that stereotyped, winning way, and not really thinking or answering." Perhaps this was a comment about the sisters' years of forced composure in the spotlight, or perhaps it was just his noticing the way the two seemed to have vacated their bodies. The psychiatrist further observed that Wilma's illness had probably been present a long time, but because she tended toward passivity, it was something she had learned to withstand without others noticing.

Edna was in and out of treatment herself, always improving at the hospital and then relapsing at home. She would have had longer stays if not for the costly bills. At home, she was very hostile toward Helen, snapping at her if she tried to bring the newspaper and even threatening to kill her for looking at her the wrong way. In May 1954, the same month the US Supreme Court made history by declaring segregation in public schools unconstitutional, the oldest sister attempted to take her own life, swallowing nine grains of sodium amytal (a sedative) and four grains of Anacin (an analgesic). Though her overdose did not render her unconscious, she was taken to the hospital.

Now it was the third daughter's turn to go crazy. Following graduation, Sarah's life had most approximated that of other twenty-somethings. She had the most respected and intellectually challenging job (at the law firm Hughes & Campbell), not to mention her notary public license. One of the attorneys she worked for was rather high-strung and cruel, often insulting her for not speaking more eloquently; still, she was happy. "I felt that I was really someone," she later recalled. "I had my own ideas and went apart from the rest of them." She joined a secretaries' club and began buying her own outfits.

But as time went on, she lost the spring in her step. Unpaid overtime wore her down, as did her father's constant oversight. Carl often interrupted club meetings to check up on her. He suspected she was really out "hounding around." He protested whenever she went with co-workers to see a "poisonous" movie, eavesdropped whenever someone phoned the house, and opened her mail, prompting her to use her office address. As in their youth, association with anyone outside their family greatly grieved him. "I don't believe he ever thought so much to what we actually were doing. It was the fact that we would get too familiar with someone."

Carl surely would have been irate to know that his wife talked to Sarah about birth control. Sadie told Sarah that she could see her doctor for more information about getting a diaphragm. Sarah listened and then, seeming to forget her father's hostility toward big families, asked if it was Sadie's use of such a device that had caused Carl to be so unloving. "I have noticed that all of my life he never seemed to have any affection for you," she confessed. Actually, replied her mother, it was Carl who was adamant about not wanting more children. She added that Sarah was not to talk about the diaphragm with Helen, who could not be trusted with the information.

Sarah casually dated a few guys behind her father's back but was soon too frightened by men to even kiss any of them. Just like Edna and Wilma, she was sexually assaulted. First, a man at work kissed her without her permission. Then a client came into the office and started talking about sex when no one else was around. He touched her arm and asked how she felt about it. When she said she was busy, he dragged her before a mirror and said, "Look at that mirror. Your eyes indicate that you are soft and can be lured into anything." He explained that she had no mind of her own and that she could never hold her own sexually—he could hypnotize her in two minutes if he wanted. She wriggled away and hurried home to tell her mother.

If mental unsoundness—or presumed mental unsoundness—made women like the Morlok quadruplets easy prey in the workplace, it also served as an excuse for their assailants' sins. When Sadie showed up at the law firm to report what had happened, one of the attorneys advised that the family not bring any charges against the fellow, as he'd been mentally ill at one point in his life. In case Sadie wasn't moved by this, he added that there were no witnesses to corroborate Sarah's story. When later interviewed about the incident, this man said it was all a figment of her imagination.

This gaslighting occurred against the backdrop of amplified exhortations to protect the gentler sex. Following the *Brown v. Board* ruling (against school segregation), the public had gone hysterical over young white women's vulnerability. In fact, knowing a ruling for the plaintiff would provoke such outcry, President Eisenhower had urged Chief Justice Earl Warren to be charitable toward segregationists, who weren't "bad people"—only parents wanting to ensure "their sweet little girls [were] not required to sit in school alongside some big black bucks." But society remained uninterested in protecting white girls and women from the predations of white men.

That night Sarah went home and took three grains of sodium amytal, sleeping until four a.m., when she woke up screaming, "Mama, help me." Her mother gave her more medicine to coax her back to sleep.

She tried to keep working, but her fears quickly intensified. As her aggressor had been wearing a brown suit, she now recoiled from all men in brown suits. When she took leave to seek outpatient psychiatric help, she struggled to tell the clinicians what had happened. Every time she talked about it, she could hear his voice. She was diagnosed with schizophrenia, undifferentiated type. As her case was not considered acute, she wasn't hospitalized.

It was a testament to Sarah's pluck—and probably also a lack of workers' rights—that she refused to let her professional skills atrophy even as she was receiving treatment. She spent many hours practicing typing in her room. The sound bothered Carl and Edna, but with all six family members in the house, it was impossible for everyone to be comfortable. There was invariably someone wanting a lamp on and another who shied at the light; someone who wanted to play the radio and another who was going down for a nap. And then there was Wilma, throwing laundry all over the lawn and pulling books off the shelves. In September, she was hospitalized with worsened symptoms. The following month, Sadie underwent a bladder surgery.

It might have been witnessing her sisters' distress that finally pushed Helen over the edge. Shortly after Edna's attempted suicide, she tried ending things herself, taking Anacin and the antihistamine neohetramine, which only gave her nausea and vomiting. She'd begun to walk off-gait, click her jaw, repeat words, and cling to her mother every waking hour. Over the summer, she stopped eating except what Sadie spoon-fed her. She trembled about darkness in broad daylight and hallucinated a great conflagration. "Oh, oh, Mama, Mama, stop it, stop it, save, save," Helen would shriek. "The fire is going to burn all of us." In December 1954, the last of the Morlok sisters was diagnosed with schizophrenia, catatonic type, and treated with electroshock.

Sadie was now at her wits' end and in pain from her operation. She hobbled about the house trying to coax one daughter to try a nap while another stirred from hers. In between bites of a hastily made sandwich, she was always trying to get someone to drink water. She could not hear herself think because Wilma was always slamming doors, and Edna was perpetually picking fights with people. Because Carl was adamant that word not spread about their troubles, he would not permit Sadie to ask for help. He did not even allow Sarah to run errands for her, fearing she would give herself away. He himself offered no assistance, still taking to the garage to bemoan the state of humanity and leaving dozens of beer bottles in his wake. He had stopped going to work altogether, though he was still drawing his pay.

Just when things were at their bleakest for Sadie, Dr. Himler suggested that the leading scientific research institution in the nation take Edna, Wilma, Sarah, and Helen off her hands. With her approval, he arranged for someone to come and see if the quadruplets were suited for study.

Sadie would later struggle to remember the days leading up to the family's journey to the East Coast, saying only that she had the sensation of being in a dark tunnel with the faintest flicker of light ahead. Maybe in her fury, she drew strength from the memory of keeping the quadruplets alive in the nursery all those years ago. Some part of her must have wandered back to the first time they'd depended upon her for everything, when her voice and touch were all. In the beginning, there'd only been love. Mother love, become flesh and multiplied. Mother love that was true and good and beautiful.

Chapter Eight

When David Rosenthal went to work for the adult psychology lab within NIMH's Clinical Center in 1955, there were few more prestigious jobs for a scientific man like him. Even the center's building conferred an air of importance, with its clean red brick, a cornerstone laid by President Truman, and its Lorraine-cross shape (one long axis cut by two shorter axes to signify the swift transfer of biomedical knowledge from the laboratories, or short axes, to the patients' bedsides in the middle).

Not only was it an honor to work for the NIMH's psychology lab—so much so that the lab could get away with paying salaries below those in academia and other industries—but researchers also had great liberties when it came to their subjects of investigation. They could take their time, too, there being no publish-or-perish mandate. These latter two factors surely attracted a man with Rosenthal's intellectual curiosity.

If someone had a particular interest in a subject, they only needed to discuss it with the lab's director Dave Shakow during their weekly meeting with him. Shakow might heartily approve, suggest an alteration, or even propose an entirely new direction. But in the words of Morris Parloff, the colleague who recommended Rosenthal for NIMH, these were "treated as collegial suggestions rather than commands." The lab's philosophy was that people had been hired on the basis of their interest and competence in a particular area, and even if their subject was high-risk, they should be given the chance to apply their talents. If working in an area that took a long time to develop, there was proper leeway to publish findings. Representatives of other NIH organizations were peeved when lab researchers were put up for promotion with scant papers in their name. "My God," some said, seeing candidates' applications, "I've got research assistants who have more publications than that."

With this liberal research climate, it was no wonder that NIMH researchers initially hoped to keep the Morlok quadruplets at the Clinical Center indefinitely, gathering data on them from as many angles as possible. While the sisters only stayed for three years, researchers would end up with far more material than Rosenthal knew what to do with when the time came to synthesize the findings, following their departure in 1958.

A few months before Rosenthal took up his post, the Morlok quadruplets had traveled via train to Bethesda, ready to undergo diagnostic tests and participate in different forms of therapy. Carl and Sadie accompanied them for the first month, then made another shorter visit. With six of the Clinical Center's twenty-four wards—a total of 150 beds—devoted to mental health research, there was space for them to periodically stay in a room adjoining the two shared by the quadruplets. (The sisters paired up as usual—Edna with Sarah, and Wilma with Helen—though it was agreed all four should eventually room with other patients.) The family was escorted from Michigan by Dr. Seymour Perlin, the psychiatrist who'd visited their home, and a nurse. Perlin had actually begun his work on the train, asking the quadruplets questions about their family life while their father was out of earshot. Perhaps he feared

Carl would change his mind before the studies got under way. Carl had been lured by the promise of free health care, both for his daughters and for himself, but that didn't mean he wouldn't revoke consent for their treatment at the drop of a hat. As Rosenthal would learn for himself, the man was incredibly suspicious of their work, and he tended to relay his suspicions to his daughters. He frequently insisted they were going to be bled to death and then go home in caskets.

Upon arriving at the Clinical Center, the quadruplets were assembled before dozens of people. Some were researchers, and others were clinicians who worked in the ward, 3-East, where the family was initially assigned to stay. These people looked them up and down, asked questions of them, and then sent them for full physical examinations. They then conferred with one another about what kind of care the sisters required and what researchers should be assigned to study the family. The Quadruplets Research Committee was formed and Parloff named to chair it.

Researchers decided that each quadruplet would have her own psychiatrist and medical doctor. That way, they'd get individualized attention, and there would be no rivalry for the experts' affections. The four psychiatrists would report to Lewis Hill, a professor at Johns Hopkins and the chief psychiatrist of Sheppard and Enoch Pratt Hospital in nearby Towson. (Hill specialized in psychotherapeutic interventions for schizophrenics, publishing a book on the topic that year.) Carl and Sadie would each have their own caseworker. When admitted to the center, they'd meet daily with this person. When in Lansing, they could communicate by phone or mail.

The sisters would not be administered hard drugs, which would corrupt the studies. In addition to psychotherapy, they'd participate in occupational therapy. It was hoped they would also benefit from the many activities and amenities that their ward and the broader campus had to offer. The ward had a small lounge with board games, books, and a piano. The Clinical Center boasted a beauty shop, newsstand, and retail store, which were frequented by researchers, clinicians, and patients alike. And if the quadruplets proved responsible, they would be permitted to wander the grounds, which had gardens and bike paths. This setup was for both investigative and therapeutic purposes. If patients lived in an environment resembling the "real" world, staff could observe them in that world and they could learn to get along in it. On 3-East, nurses and other aides were expected to record observations of patients' behaviors and social interactions, which researchers like the ward's administrator, Murray Bowen, studied to better understand the mentally ill and their families.

There was something else that NIMH offered the Morlok quadruplets: people like them. For the first time in their lives, they were surrounded by multiples, at least some of whom had a serious mental illness. There was one triplet who showed a particular interest in them, assuring Sarah and Edna that they didn't ever have to put on a show for him.

The members of the Quadruplets Research Committee were slower in forging connections. As the committee was so vast, eventually exceeding thirty people, there were many disparate opinions and personalities, along with confusion about who exactly was therapeutically responsible for the Morloks. Everyone seemed to regard the family as a shared research object—there for any and all to utilize in their respective projects. Parloff found it so difficult to work with certain people, as well as to supervise the whole lot, that when Rosenthal came on board, he happily surrendered the reins to the one he'd suggested for hire. Perhaps this was his plan all along, although he offered a different rationale for the change of guard when speaking with documentarians years later: Not only did Rosenthal have greater expertise on schizophrenia, but his temperament was better suited for the role. He was warm in his own quiet way, and people couldn't help but admire him. "He had great patience and could deal well with all of the people involved." His management style was to listen carefully to what everyone had to say and then follow his original hunch. "As a result, he spent less time in meetings and more time getting things done."

Rosenthal's own first meeting with the quadruplets was never recounted. One can only wonder what he thought as he beheld them for the first time or what words passed between them. But he would later record some observations of the family. Carl was "dejected, tense, and ill at ease," but too meek to relay complaints except through his wife. Generally, he "seemed almost unable to do anything without first checking with his wife." No doubt, this impression proved incomplete when Rosenthal learned from reading Carl's chart that, finding himself unable to express his criticisms directly to staff, he'd attempted to choke Sadie in the privacy of their room.

Sadie was "pleasant, sociable, and amiable." She was clearly the one to take charge of the family, seeing that all were well groomed, fed, rested, and sufficiently active. She was "always ready to help any of them who needed it, her husband included." But her misgivings about their being at the center were evident. She often doubted whether she'd done the right thing in bringing the quadruplets, once asking if it was possible for people to die from unhappiness. She grew especially morose whenever the time came for her to return home with Carl. The last week of their original stay, she'd complained of headache, weakness, nausea, hot flashes, and tightness all over. She was too helpless even to brush her teeth, having to implore the staff for help. One day a nurse found her lying in bed, kicking her feet. When asked what was wrong, she could only say, "Oh, things are just so awful. I feel so ill and weak. I never felt this way before. I feel so strange."

The quadruplets were surprisingly distinct. Edna struck Rosenthal as quiet, compliant, slow-spoken, and withdrawn. She sometimes appeared to be hallucinating. Wilma was thin, fragile, and frightened. She often stood motionless, but would giggle in response to her own hallucinations. Sarah was the most friendly, pleasant, and talkative of the bunch, though she, too, was clearly under great strain. She may have gotten a little carried away by the comforts at the Clinical Center, calling nurses into her room to wait on her and then saying, "That's all for now." Helen was totally out of touch with reality. Fearing that fires were always edging closer and closer, she constantly wanted someone by her side. All were initially diagnosed with schizophrenic reaction, catatonic type. (In Michigan, only Helen had been found to have this type, the other three appearing to be "undifferentiated.")

Taking the four troubled sisters together, Rosenthal was overwhelmed by a sense of their significance to psychiatric genetics. In his own words, he "could hardly help but wonder what further proof of a genetic etiology of schizophrenia anyone would want to have." His mind turned to Bénédict Augustin (Auguste) Morel, the French psychiatrist who'd first tried to articulate a theory of inheritance nearly one hundred years before. After visiting mental asylums across Europe and studying patients' family history and childhood experiences, Morel had postulated that a family started with a nervous temperament, which then developed in the next generation with cerebral hemorrhages, idiopathic affections of the brain, and neuroses. By the third generation, the disposition toward insanity and dangerous acts was innate; and by the fourth, there was sterility, idiocy, and cretinous degeneration. Morel's idea that the insane would naturally become sterile had never taken off, but his concept of hereditary tainting remained compelling and not just among those with eugenicist inclinations.

The more Rosenthal came to know the family's history, however, the more it became apparent that the Morloks did not so neatly illustrate Morel's theory, nor that of any other psychiatric geneticist. Their case was more useful for considering the relation between life experiences and outcomes where heredity was controlled, and the types of hereditarian or environmental factors that might be implicated. As he'd clarify in his book, some experts assumed that a single, mutant gene constituted nature's contribution, while others believed schizophrenics inherited multiple mutant genes of individually small effect. For some, the constitutional predisposition could be as vague as personality defects, roundabout ways of thinking, or a conglomeration of behavioral patterns. On the nurture side, there was disagreement about whether schizophrenics were victims of some prenatal factor, a failure of cognitive integration, a failure of socialization, a failure to contain anxiety, or something else. With such varied opinions, it was essential to engage researchers from all different disciplines in studying the Morloks.

To apprehend the hereditarian factors at play, investigators needed to study the maternal and paternal lines, confirm that the quadruplets were in fact monozygotic (by testing their blood, analyzing their fingerprints, and considering Sadie's placenta), and take other anatomical measurements of all six members of the family. DNA testing did not yet exist, but there were diagnostics such as electroencephalography (EEG), which measured electrical activity, and galvanic skin response tests, which measured the electrical characteristics of the skin in response to auditory and visual stimuli. Rosenthal and his colleagues believed these could help them to approximate the ways in which the quadruplets anatomically favored one parent over the other, as well as to make other inferences about their inheritance.

When it came to psychological and environmental influences, they could go well beyond psychiatric interviews, utilizing doll play, draw-a-person tests, Rorschach protocols, and more. They could even send sociologists to Lansing to interview the quadruplets' teachers, neighbors, and associates. To the best of Rosenthal's knowledge, these people were unaware that the quadruplets were suffering from any mental illness, and he was not inclined to give them away. When he wrote to request interviews on behalf of his colleagues, he only revealed that the sisters were being studied "as part of [NIMH's] research on the social and personal problems of families with multiple births and on the process of personality development."

Although absorbed with this work of mapping the Morlok family—biologically, psychologically, socially—Rosenthal was soon persuaded to take on additional research at the Patuxent Institution, a newly opened maximum-security prison in Jessup, Maryland, that provided psychotherapeutic treatment to inmates. He went to Patuxent on Thursdays, then worked Saturdays at NIMH to make up for the lost hours. There weren't researchers going in and out of the ward on the weekends, so he could visit the quadruplets without fear of disrupting any important business.

His children would come to take far more interest in his prison work, especially after he came home with a bandaged arm after being attacked by an inmate. The side gig also helped to make ends meet. Even with his wife collecting savings stamps, sewing her own clothes, and perpetually comparing grocery prices between Safeway and A&P, they had to stretch to pay all the bills. But it wasn't as though the family wanted for anything. Rosenthal's son Scott fondly remembers "going out to eat" at the NIH cafeteria, climbing the jungle gyms on the campus, visiting the capital monuments, and having liberty to roam the neighborhood until the streetlights came on. All the residents' yards backed up to a field, where there was nearly always a game of football going.

Perhaps a great reason for the family's merriment was that his father never brought his work home with him. In fact, it would be many years before Scott understood the gravity of his father's research on mental illness. Only ever seeing the man who loved jokes and helping with math homework, he never thought to ask if it was psychologically or emotionally wearing to engage with people whose struggles were so severe. He does know, though, that his father tended not to view perpetrators of harm—not even the most violent criminals at Patuxent—as evil. His scientific training inclined him to see such people as pathological.

Carl Morlok proved no exception. Given the chance to make sense of the man who'd so terrorized his own children, Rosenthal approached the infamous Lansing constable with more curiosity than judgment. So did his colleagues. And as happened so often in psychiatric cases, they found a deeply wounded soul. Someone who seemed to have drawn a very bad lot and who'd been tormented long before he became a tormentor.

Chapter Nine

On the day he was born, Carl's mother went out in the field and flailed grain, hoping to abort him. Before that, Katherine Morlok had tried to induce a miscarriage by cleaning stables and lifting heavy things. She wanted nothing more than for a dead baby to come out of her. She hadn't wanted to be pregnant after the sixth child, resenting her husband for impregnating her twice more. During both of these pregnancies (not even her last), she'd threatened to kill Gottlieb Morlok for what he'd done.

Gottlieb felt he had to keep a close eye on his wife to see that she didn't try anything brazen. Rumor had it she'd gone nuts for three years during her teens. Not only was Katherine erratic, she was manipulative. She often faked coughing spells and even heart attacks to keep him from smoking. Her husband always knew she was acting, but, like Sadie witnessing her "seizures" in the years to come, he never let on. That would only have made her angrier.

Years later, once they'd moved from the German village of Metzingen to America, she'd bribe her children to exert control. She paid Carl twenty-five cents to stay home from a Fourth of July celebration. His loyalty was to be toward the mother country. Carl probably didn't need the money to comply, as he always feared something terrible befalling Katherine. Once when he took an extended trip with his brother, he could not quiet his thoughts of catastrophe back home.

Gottlieb, for his part, was not exactly a stable parent. He drank heavily and got ugly under the influence. Both he and Katherine threatened Carl and his siblings with mental illness if they ever masturbated. They also let on that it was better to die than to be insane.

If Carl grew up under the shadow of being unwanted, he was also haunted by a ghost. His immediately elder sister had died at only two months old under mysterious circumstances. She was thought to be a little off. But if anyone ever inquired about the manner of the infant's death, his family acted strange, offering no explanation.

In addition to this specter, the future father of the quadruplets had a stutter, and he knew well enough to hate himself for it. Whenever words got caught in his throat, he swelled with loathing until he could force them out. But he early learned to project his disgust onto enemy bodies. America had long affirmed open season on Blacks, and his people had a special revulsion to Jews; thus, he psychologically exploited both. These two hatreds had historically come in a pair. Long before Hitler declared Jews a "negroid parasite on the national body," both Western Christianity and science had put Jews and Blacks together. In the Christian imagination, the two were darkened by their turning away from God. In the secular imagination, the two had turned away from reason.

By the time Carl arrived at NIMH, many experts had begun to wonder if existential anxieties undergirded racism. Perhaps the white man's fear of death caused him to see the racialized other as half dead. Perhaps the anti-Semite's perception of his own porous body made him regard the Jew as fleshy and feminine. Or maybe infantile tendencies best explained human bigotry. The Swiss American psychoanalyst Richard Sterba decided so when, following the 1943 race riot in Detroit, his white patients in the city reported dreams of beheading, hunting, and aborting Black people. In Sterba's mind, such violent images evidenced a combination of Oedipal conflicts and sibling rivalry.

By reframing racism as psychological conflict, experts like Sterba seemed to believe, they could bring all of a person's problems under the purview of science. This way of thinking was at least as old as psychoanalysis. Wanting his program to be taken seriously—to be taken as *science*—Freud had long encouraged "evenly hovering listening." Analysts were never to bring their politics into the room, nor to resort to political explanations for their patients' psychic woes. Rather, they were to act as blank screens onto which analysands could project ("transfer") all their fears and desires.

It might seem that the Holocaust would weaken this tradition of neutrality, seeing as it meant an astounding number of people were mental cases. In fact, it fortified it. Hitler became known as a "madman" and Germany, a "paranoid" nation. Even those directly traumatized by Nazism adopted the morally impartial language of pathology. When Jewish analysts fled to the US, they did not speak of what they'd endured and, instead, determined to be the disembodied listeners that America mandated for its own victims and perpetrators of racism. "It simply didn't matter if a case had its roots in the Holocaust or that a patient or their parent had survived atrocity," scholar of psychoanalysis Hannah Zeavin has written of the postwar therapeutic landscape. "All that mattered was the transference, the psychic action in the room."

It was probably partly because the "psy" professions were decidedly *not* looking for Nazis that Rosenthal and other NIMH investigators made no note of Carl being one, instead considering the possibility that he was mentally ill. It surely didn't hurt that his family history supported this hypothesis, nor that Carl struck so many staff as being more pitiable than tyrannizing. Nor that NIMH's ranks included no Black psychiatrists or psychologists, who were far less willing, in Zeavin's words, to "bracket the world" when considering individuals' woes. Whatever their reasons, the NIMH researchers looked past Carl's hatred, closing the door on sociological inquiries just as many Freudians had done before them.

Sadie was the first to recount Carl's dysfunctional upbringing, along with his many troubled relatives. In Rosenthal's words, she presented the Morlok family as "abounding with various forms of psychopathology" and her own clan as nearly free of mental disorders. Of course this stark contrast had raised questions about her credibility, but Carl's brother John confirmed many of her claims. One of Carl's uncles was known to be psychotic, and his eldest brother, Bill, was a "moron type." This brother, the one whose wife had professed love for Carl all those years ago, had once been found in bed with his thirteen-year-old daughter. The girl herself was believed to be disordered and was compelled to have her tubes tied. Bill also had a son who had a cleft palate and tied tongue, which many took as signs of his own imbecility. There was a cousin who'd masturbated in public and been deported back to Germany. Then there was the interviewed brother, John. According to Sadie, he heard voices and had a breakdown upon his daughter's marriage at twenty-five. He'd cried and wandered about, saying how he'd only ever lived to see her marry and make a nice home. Now that she had, he didn't know if his life had any meaning.

Carl appeared to be similarly vulnerable. In sessions with his caseworker, he spoke tenderly of all of his daughters except Helen. ("She's as ornery as ever and is the worst of the bunch," he said.) In fact, he was so lonesome for his children that he began to accuse NIMH staff of trying to wean his daughters off him and keep them indefinitely. To this, his caseworker replied that mentally ill people often required professional help and his daughters would need his support when they came out of the hospital. Furthermore, all children eventually left the family circle. It was just a part of life. Carl seemed to appreciate these words.

While Carl complimented his own fathering, he made a point to emphasize that his wife had done the bulk of the parenting. According to his caseworker, he "took almost no credit for the part he played in the early rearing of the girls and stated that the father's primary responsibility to a family was in making a living for them." He simply would not tolerate anyone thinking of him in effeminate terms. He much preferred to talk about his job, which gave him feelings of self-importance. He spent many hours telling stories that highlighted his duties as constable. He also tended to disclose unflattering details about himself or his daughters only through these anecdotes. For instance, he claimed to meet many alcoholics on the job, finding that they were "misunderstood" or victims of circumstances beyond their control. Was this his way of pleading for sympathy for his own addiction? His caseworker sure wondered. Carl also told of a person who was once blamed for something awful that was really not his fault. Asked pointedly if this compared to his getting blamed for his daughters' illnesses, he lowered his head and mumbled something about people not understanding what it was like to be the father of quadruplets.

Time and again, Carl stressed that he was a good father. "I can't understand why the girls are sick," he'd say. "I have done all I could to make a good home for them. I used to take them to church; they are good Christians. I spent a great deal of money on their care." Sometimes he blamed overwork as the cause of their decline. Other times, he sighed and cited God's will.

His caseworker characterized Carl as having a "depressive quality... accentuated by a spiritless, slowly paced walk" and "a preference to remain in the background." Overall Carl seemed like "a small-town factory hand," who wanted to please people in his own awkward way. He often brought sample packages of cigarettes he'd gotten from someone at the Red Cross, handing them over "like a schoolboy offering his teacher an apple." So smitten was his caseworker that he didn't even seem to take offense when Carl, startled to learn that he was Jewish, said, "Well, there's good and bad in all of us."

Some might say this was the alchemy of the therapeutic space, the way it drew out the gentleness in people. But what did it mean for those outside the room when a person's more violent tendencies receded from view? What was it going to mean for the quadruplet studies that the sisters' primary abuser was now being compared to a tenderhearted schoolboy?

Sadie corroborated that Carl was an increasingly helpless man, further domesticating the longtime tormentor even if that was not her intention. She told, for instance, how her husband was deeply humiliated by his impotence. Back at home, he'd try to get into bed with her only to say, "I'm just getting you all worked up so you'll have to go out to some hound to take care of you." Carl still tried to be a despot. If she did not turn the light off promptly by nine o'clock, he'd accuse her of "lying in [her] nakedness" and flirting with some man outside the house. But his threats didn't pack the same punch as before.

Sadie told her own caseworker she considered leaving Carl, but he was too invalid to care for himself. She'd noticed he'd begun to click his jaw just as Helen had before she'd spiraled out of control.

She felt obligated to care for him, not least because the quadruplets would deteriorate were anything bad to happen to him. Though she didn't say so, Sadie might also have savored how the tables had turned. According to one physician, she delighted in relating how unattractive she found Carl. She claimed to have only married him because his family members misrepresented him to her, adding, "He certainly has done nothing to make me love him since."

During Carl and Sadie's visits to the Clinical Center, many staff members witnessed just how pathetic Carl's efforts to dominate his wife were. They saw, for instance, how whenever Sadie had an appointment with a caseworker or some other person, he would wander the ward looking for her. If he happened to know what room she occupied, he'd pace outside and press his ear against the door. One nurse overheard him say he intended to bring his gun and shoot Dr. Perlin, whom he accused of sleeping with Sadie. (Not long after the Jewish psychiatrist had visited Sadie's room, Carl found her administering a vaginal douche, taking it as proof they'd been intimate.) There were a few staff members who were so frightened by his threats that they refused to interact with him, but most seemed to think him more bark than bite.

For their own amusement, it seems, staff sometimes exposed Carl's manipulations. After a seeming blackout spell in the hallway, a doctor determined that the incident was not epileptic in nature, as some assumed, but more likely due to a voluntary interruption of circulation in the brain. Noting that Carl's face had been flushed, not pale, while he lay on the floor, this doctor claimed that Carl had hypersensitive carotid sinuses on both sides of his neck, allowing for cardiac asystole to be produced at will by applying pressure on either side. In other words, Carl had induced the spell.

Before long, Carl's caseworker developed a theory to explain his troubles: He had been subjected to horrific parenting. In this professional's words, reminiscent of Frieda Fromm-Reichmann's schizophrenogenic mother, he was "dominated by a selfish, irascible mother, who demanded that her children care for her but met their efforts with hostile rebukes and further demands." Throughout his childhood and adolescence, he had a conflicting sense of identity. He "was either passive and retiring like his father or demanding and abusive like his mother." As a result, his male identity suffered. He never developed adequate self-esteem. The birth of the quadruplets only further emasculated him. It called into question his ability to financially provide for his children on his own, and he responded by "taking a restrictive, punishing attitude toward them under the guise of 'raising them to be good Christians.'" It didn't help that his identity had also been reduced to that of the father of the quadruplets, rather than a person in his own right.

Rosenthal was beginning to wonder if both Carl and Katherine were borderline schizophrenics, their peculiarities resembling those of people before they went psychotic. He was likely not surprised, then, when other researchers uncovered what seemed to be greater evidence of paternal influence in the foursome. Electroencephalographic studies revealed that all the sisters and Carl had occipital slow waves, which had a higher incidence in schizophrenic persons, whereas Sadie did not. And both father and daughters, but not mother, experienced childhood enuresis (involuntary urination), introversion, fatigue, and other alleged early indicators of mental illness. Two experts further deduced that Carl had some mild brain damage, based upon his performances on visual-motor and psychological tests. These findings didn't mean Sadie had played no part in genetically predisposing the quadruplets to mental illness. Polygenic (multiple gene) theories held that non-schizophrenic parents could carry some pathological genes, though not enough to be clinically schizophrenic themselves. Perhaps Sadie had passed on such genes, which combined with Carl's to provide a "constitutional host" for illness in the quadruplets.

But when it came to Sadie, mothering and personality problems most captured investigators' attention, seeming to show that no matter the profession's commitment to neutrality, prejudices *always* worked their way into diagnostic formulations. Practically echoing the child psychiatrist in Lansing, Sadie's own caseworker noted that she was "clearly thriving on the attention she received" at the Clinical Center. This professional also described Sadie as being starved for affection and having few inner resources for happiness, despite coming across as self-assured. Sadie used all sorts of classic defense mechanisms, including repression, avoidance, denial, and projection. She totally disavowed sexual feelings in herself and projected them onto male relatives or her youngest daughter.

Having decided that she was a neurotic mess, the caseworker was utterly unconvinced when Sadie reported that her husband, father, and maternal grandfather were all sexually promiscuous, each causing women to become pregnant illegitimately. It was as if the simple fact of her idiosyncrasies disproved that men were lustful. This wasn't even the worst example of female pathology overshadowing male impropriety. The social worker also expressed doubt over Sadie's claims that the quadruplets disliked Carl because of his overbearing ways. "One can surmise that mother did not control her expression of anger and resentment toward father and that this in turn made it next to impossible for the girls to express any warm feelings which they may have had for father," she wrote in Sadie's file.

Freud's female hysterics had undergone the very same gaslighting. By virtue of being hysterical, they could not possibly be taken at their word and so everything they alleged was de facto untrue. Perhaps this pattern suggests another reason why some felt compelled to pathologize bigotry: In reducing hate to mental quirk, they could effectively erase hate from the sane world. They could wave away the reality that, in terms of his attitudes toward the "inferior" classes, someone like Carl Morlok was all too normal.

If midcentury psychoanalysts and social workers permitted mothers one benefit, it was having been poorly mothered themselves. In line with this, Sadie's caseworker described her childhood as totally lacking in maternal nurturing, only secondarily mentioning Sadie's father's failings. Because her mother was constantly birthing children, this caseworker theorized, Sadie had been forced to become prematurely responsible for her younger siblings. She was also obliged to look out for her mother, who, in addition to being perpetually pregnant, was tormented by her husband. Sadie never had the chance to be mothered herself. It was no wonder that she left home at a young age, nor that she associated pregnancy with helplessness. In marriage and motherhood, her anxieties intensified, and "her use of denial and projection went beyond the usual neurotic mechanisms." She mothered Carl exactly as she would have liked to be. She washed his face, soaked his feet, and trimmed the hair in his ears, all the while saying, "It's better this way…he is not capable of doing things for himself." At the same time, she feared him as she'd once feared her father, admitting, "He is a little better to me if I look after him." She neglected and resented certain daughters exactly as she had once been neglected and resented. She had particular antipathy for Helen, whose infanthood she once summed up with the words "cry, cry, cry."

As the quadruplets aged, the caseworker elaborated, Sadie imparted her wifely responsibilities to her two most stable daughters. Edna took pains to appease Carl as Sadie had done for her father on behalf of her passive and withdrawn mother. Sarah found ways to keep the peace while privately resenting Carl. "It was as though different facets of Mrs. Morlok's unresolved childhood conflicts with her father were assigned to the two daughters to be acted out by them with their own father."

In a broader sense, she bequeathed each of her daughters with an aspect of her flawed personality. Rather than regarding them as individuals, she treated each as an extension of herself. "The girls, in turn, devoted themselves to living out the mother's mandates and thus sacrificed their own personalities." According to the caseworker, referring to Sarah, Edna, Wilma, and Helen respectively, "The 'favored' daughter was to be completely dependent upon Mother and enveloped in a symbiotic relationship with her; the second was to live out Mother's independent strivings; the third was to repress her instinctual drives as Mother strove to do; and the fourth was the embodiment of the 'bad' drives which Mother denied and assailed." It was no surprise, then, that "in her psychosis, each girl caricatured the role her mother assigned to her."

As with his own caseworker, Carl was almost entirely off the hook, his role defined only in relation to Sadie's. In her words, he "had little to offer his daughters that would remedy or dilute the mother's influence on them." Consequently, he "reinforced her pathological influence." His dependence upon Sadie increased her denial of her own unmet dependency needs, which she reassigned to Edna and Sarah. Similarly, his "sexual unsureness of himself aggravated her own sexual distortions, a central problem which she transferred to Wilma and Helen."

If this caseworker had interviewed the quadruplets, would she have come to a different conclusion? All four told of being variously tormented by Carl and aching for Sadie. Or was the impulse to mother-blame simply too strong for her to see what damage fathers could do?

Several of the five blind consultants looped into the studies were also on the hunt for an overanxious mother, all the while presenting anxiety as the product of abstract, psychodynamic forces—never as the product of religious or racial commitments. When Sadie and Carl agreed to participate in Rorschach tests, one outside evaluator knowing nothing about the family declared Sadie to be more "sexually and anally preoccupied" than Carl on the seeming basis that she saw so many "hemorrhoids, virgin female organs, and vaginal dilations" in the ink blots, while he betrayed a vaguer sense of the way people and things were "permeable and enterable." (Carl saw many blots as being the same, also using speech that suggested "amorphousness" between himself and others.) What did it mean, Sadie's sexual fixation and Carl's horror of the spilling-over body? For the test evaluator, namely that any offspring of theirs were apt to be "bodily preoccupied" and have "poor ego boundaries," which, in turn, disposed them toward schizophrenic thoughts and behaviors.

Another expert—a research psychologist—blindly evaluated Carl's responses to a Parental Attitude Research Instrument and chalked his extreme regard for masculine strength up to "authoritarian personality," a construct newly developed to explain fascism in psychoanalytic terms. The Morlok patriarch answered "strongly agree" to the following statements, among others: "The biggest mistake a man can make is marrying a woman who always wants to wear the pants of the family"; "The old-fashioned family was best because the wife kept in her place"; "Some children are just so bad they must be taught to fear adults for their own good"; "Children shouldn't be confused by letting them learn things which differ from what their parents told them"; and "A parent should never be made to look wrong in a child's eyes." Attempting to make sense of his higher-than-average preference for domination, the psychologist cited a paper explaining how feelings of personal inadequacy inclined individuals to over-control external situations. In essence, he rationalized Carl's never-named Nazism.

By repeatedly framing Carl and Sadie's "eccentricities" in terms of developmental failures, many of the investigators tacitly conveyed something about the nature of psychic violence such as theirs: It was instinctive. If this was true—if the psychic exploitation of others largely stemmed from internal drives shared by all human beings—was it possible to ever rid the world of racism such as Carl's? Would there always be autocratic mothers?

This was the dead end of Freudian psychoanalysis, according to some of the discipline's Black critics. It could heal individuals, but it could not remake the world. The founder himself had seemed to concede this point when he famously disagreed with Albert Einstein about the possibility of a civilization without war. War, in Freud's schema, was an expression of the death instinct, which was about as old as humanity. The problem with this, for critics like psychiatrist Alexander Thomas and psychologist Samuel Sillen, was that it did not explain why some countries incessantly went to war while others managed to avoid it. It was utter defeatism to pretend realities like peace and Black liberation were contingent upon certain people's emancipation from the id. The question psychiatry really needed to ask was how internal and external forces interacted—how, say, the authoritarian personality collided with Jim Crow America.

The caseworkers and researchers studying Carl and Sadie may not have thought much beyond universal instincts and mother wounds, but that was a small portion of the research team. Many more were assigned to evaluate the quadruplets, and these individuals could not possibly reduce them to these data points, at least not without totally disregarding the possibility of male violence. They were bolstered by a flowering of research on the families of schizophrenics in the mid-1950s. One in-house psychologist, Lyman Wynne, was interested in a phenomenon he called pseudo-mutuality, where a family had an appearance of harmony and understanding, but relationships were actually quite rigid and depersonalizing. He was also intrigued by the "rubber fence" family, which was so insular that when outsiders wanted in or members wanted out, they "sprang back tightly."

Far more pressing to the quadruplets than scientific explanations, however, was the matter of their recovery. They had not come to NIMH to understand what was wrong with them or their parents, but to be made new. Even with people circling in and out of the ward to collect information about her, one of the sisters was managing to enter the exhilarating worlds of dream and play, where so many others had come face-to-face with their fears. But it was psychotherapy that Sarah would always remember for helping her back to her body. On the couch, finding her *own* words, she was reborn.

Chapter Ten

Sarah enters a room. A woman shows her to a table, where miniature dolls sit: twenty-six rubber human figures, including a policeman, doctor, nurse, priest, and civilians of all ages. There's dining and living room furniture, too. The woman, who is a psychologist, explains that Sarah is to put on a stage production. She should make it as dramatic as possible and narrate everything she's doing. Sarah smiles and nods nervously, then looks at the dolls. "They're dressed so cute," she says in a voice that strikes one observer as excessively saccharine.

Unbeknownst to her, Rosenthal and research psychologist Blanche Usdansky, who knows nothing about Sarah's family history, are watching the proceedings through a one-way mirror. They're also audio-recording her remarks so that Usdansky, one of the hired consultants, can more carefully analyze them. Though doll play has only sparingly been used with psychotic adults—it was developed in the early century to elicit conflicts, identifications, defense mechanisms, and psychic preoccupations in children—these two experts believe it will prove helpful in understanding the interior worlds of the quadruplets.

"Um, I'm not too good at this, I don't think," Sarah mumbles. She picks up a couch and then a rocker. She runs her finger across other furniture before tentatively arranging the pieces into something resembling a living room. "You don't mind what I set up here?" she asks. The psychologist reminds her there are no parameters to the content. "When I was younger, I didn't have anything like this to play with," she says.

She struggles to get going, again double-checking the rules: "Now should I tell you what I have in mind or what?" The woman says yes. A moment later, Sarah asks her to confirm a basic object. "This is a table, right?" Usdansky can already sense that she is an extremely anxious person.

Sarah picks up a policeman, leading the observing psychologist to wonder if she is searching for control. She then sets the figure down and goes for an adult woman. She sets this down, too, and retrieves a small boy and girl. These, she seems to decide, are safer. She plays with their limbs and tries to get them to stand. Then she has them dance, as if to the music of a phonograph or television in the room. She adds another couple to the dance floor, explaining, "More than one couple on the floor looks better." She laughs nervously. "My imagination isn't very good."

The psychologist in the room praises her on her work so far. Seemingly buoyed, Sarah goes for an adult male figure, putting him before the dancing couple. "He might be around." Usdansky wonders if she is expressing guilt for her romantic scene or perhaps a wish for a chaperone figure.

She introduces a lady, saying this might be an older sister or mother. She then sits a small girl in an armchair and another off to the side. Now the scene approximates her own family. There are four girls, one woman, and one man—plus the two boy dancing partners. At this point, the psychologist asks for a story. Sarah is sheepish but offers some thoughts. The man is "a supervisor, maybe...to keep the children from doing the kind of things you know they want to." The woman is "doing what she can to make it successful and serving nourishments and party favors." As for the two girls sitting on the sidelines, "They are waiting on the next dance or helping out the others." Perhaps intuiting how closely art is imitating life, she retreats from the whole charade. "I think that's about as much as I can do," she says.

The psychologist presses her to continue, reminding her to be dramatic. Sarah suggests there may be tension between the girls. Perhaps one of those sitting to the side is jealous that the boy keeps dancing with the same girl. This hypothetical seems to make her so guilty she can't even state it firmly.

After this, the psychologist asks her to put on a children's show. It's all part of the investigative procedure, though she doesn't say so. Once again Sarah goes for the furniture first. Perhaps, thinks Usdansky, this is a sign that she seeks safety in the impersonal, approaching relationships with more caution. Sarah arranges the inanimate objects into a hospital scene, then selects a child. She's having "her tonsils taken out or something." These last two words transfix Usdansky. Perhaps "or something" means a more invasive procedure, signaling some sort of castration anxiety?

Sarah has the nurse and doctor come check on the child patient. Then she makes the doctor lean over the patient, as if he is trying to closely examine her. "Whoops. You're going to be over there in the bed with her," she says of the figure, who can't be bent at the waist. Having uttered what sounds to Usdansky like an Oedipal wish, she is mortified. She tries backpedaling, mumbling about the cuteness of the figures. Then, for whatever reason, she proceeds with the taboo thought: "I think he wants to go right to bed with her." She lays the doctor down next to the girl, then sits the nurse in a nearby chair. She gathers other girl figures and places them around the scene, saying they "are so excited about this one in the bed... wondering what's going to happen next." So is Usdansky. Will it be a tonsillectomy or sex?

Sarah knows she's gone too far, reverting to nervousness once more. She says that she is worried about breaking the dolls. Then she announces a third production, one that will be more suited for children. It involves kids following behind a policeman to cross a street on their way to school. One of the girls tells a boy she is going to beat him there, spurring the boy to make a mad dash across the street. He is badly injured by an oncoming car, and his mother screams. The cop calls for an ambulance. Usdansky wonders if she is making some comment about male competitiveness and perhaps another about female ineffectuality.

After this, the psychologist leaves the room, and Sarah is left alone. This, too, is part of the script. She picks up the nurse and gazes at her for a few moments. Then she puts her alongside the doctor. They embrace. She next lines up all the little girl dolls as if they are a trail of little ducklings. She looks around, unsure if anyone is watching, and puts the infant in the nurse's arms. The sequence strikes Usdansky as more deviant than any of the others. Here, she has allowed the idea of sex to come to full fruition.

Sarah suddenly turns to the mirror. Does she see them? For a moment, it seems so, but then she simply pats her hair into place. The session soon concludes, and the tape recorder is stopped.

When Usdansky later reflected on Sarah's doll play, she couldn't help but note certain persistent themes: the presence of chaperones, the preference for nonhuman objects, the deep curiosity about sex. She was also struck by the "stereotyped quality" of Sarah's remarks.

In her words, Sarah's productions were "like a ritualized enactment of a doll-like child's performance for the ladies in the living room visiting Mother, a well-rehearsed effort to please." It wasn't just any mother whom Sarah appeared eager to satisfy, but a mother out of Frieda Fromm-Reichmann's imagination. Though she had no knowledge of the quadruplets' familial history, Usdansky went so far as to say that Sarah sounded "a bit like the schizophrenogenic mother when talking to her child in front of strangers." Having made this connection, she proceeded to insult the spied-upon woman. In reference to Sarah's "exaggeratedly apologetic quality," Usdansky claimed to be reminded "of some masochists, whose excessive 'don't hit me' air is in itself irritating to other people and likely to invite punishment."

Edna, Wilma, and Helen had their own turns at doll play, though none of the three executed the command to tell a story, providing Usdansky with far less content to analyze. Edna struck the psychologist as being vacant and withdrawn. Wilma was more animated, sometimes even "psychotic-looking." Helen gave the impression she was hallucinating, laughing to herself and then dully staring into space.

Edna was more cooperative with draw-a-person tests, which were conducted to provide insight into their more latent self-conceptions. Psychologist Isabelle V. Kendig visited the ward several times and asked them to draw both a man and woman, then analyzed their sketches without any knowledge of their history. (Wilma and Helen only participated in one round.) According to this outside expert, Sarah's women were satisfactorily feminine but conveyed possible feelings of inadequacy with their hands behind their backs. Edna's women were stiff, suggesting underlying aggression or perhaps some confusion over sexual roles. Wilma's one woman was virtually indistinguishable from her man, suggesting "extreme" confusion over such roles. Helen was the only sister to draw a man first, signaling "uncertainty of her own gender." Even more notably, both of Helen's figures' hands reached toward their genitals—a sure sign of "sexual preoccupation," as far as the interpreter was concerned. It doesn't appear that Kendig considered memories of sexual abuse.

Blindly analyzing Rorschach protocols collected from the sisters, psychologist Margaret Thaler Singer found that all four took after their father and showed a fixation "with disease, dirt, and being intruded." Sarah and Helen also identified religious content in the ink, suggesting an additional preoccupation with the spiritual realm. Helen described hatchets, a sword, an arrow, a burning bush, a fire, a tornado, and "the walls of Jerusalem [sic] tumbling down." Perhaps because religious-themed delusions had long been observed in paranoid schizophrenics, these tropes did not strike Singer as particularly significant. Another psychologist who blindly evaluated Rorschach protocols—in this case, for diagnostic purposes—also observed religious fixations in Sarah and Helen but attributed them to an "epileptic" personality. (In his mind, their "preoccupation with violence," especially their "fear of becoming a victim of aggression," was further suggestive of seizure disorder.)

Thea Stein Lewinson, a handwriting analyst, evaluated samples of the sisters' pre- and post-diagnosis writing for personality and psychopathology. Knowing only that her subjects were schizophrenic quadruplets, Lewinson also identified "religious attachments" and "strict, fundamental moral principles" in the quadruplets. In her formulation, these provided them with the "moral support" they could not muster from within. Lewinson noted "idiosyncrasies," "inner blocks," "infantile" emotions, "hypersensitive" tendencies, and "aggressive tendencies [that came] to the surface." In her mind, as well, then, the quadruplets' problems had little to do with anything that had happened *to* them; they were an effect of their being so "badly equipped to meet internal or external crises."

The NIMH staff who personally interacted with the quadruplets were more generous. The ward workers, especially, seemed to understand how much power their parents wielded with their words and deeds. Around twenty-five staff members recorded observations of familial interactions, many relating to Carl's efforts to surveil the quadruplets or Sadie's coldness toward Helen. These staff members were not given any specific instructions, nor asked to be comprehensive with their documentation. One, presumably a nurse, described Carl interrupting as she gave Edna an enema, adding, "I don't believe I have spent more than a few moments in a room at a time with any member of the family when Mr. Morlok hasn't come in." The collected observations were turned over to a psychologist to make meaning of them.

If NIMH researchers had their prejudices, they were also fearful of bias, supposing that the less people knew about the family when reviewing a set of data, the more scientific their findings. Rosenthal later explained that it was also a matter of wanting to have disparate points of view. "Our concern was not to see if test analyses would yield diagnoses that matched [those] based on psychiatric interviews and observations. Rather, we hoped that the test would yield information in its own right." And there *were* NIMH investigators looking holistically at the family, some by rather unconventional means. In addition to interviewing people in Lansing, a sociologist named Olive Quinn was studying the collection of family scrapbooks (the "looking glass") and the extensive media coverage of the family. She was beginning to understand the quadruplets' problems as resulting from their inability to differentiate themselves from one another or develop an ego.

Lyman Wynne suspected such "confusion of experience within the family," combined with their "almost complete lack of experience" beyond the family, produced illness. In a paper presented at the 1957 International Congress of Psychiatry while the quadruplets were still at NIMH, he further claimed their case cast doubt on the theory that schizophrenia of insidious onset in childhood or early adolescence was predominantly hereditary, while schizophrenia of more acute and transient forms was predominantly environmental. Citing the sisters' markedly different roles within the family and their disparate clinical presentations, he posited that one's place in the family structure could shape the course of disease.

The communications scholar Gregory Bateson and several of his colleagues furnished investigators with another theory to consider: Schizophrenia resulted from an ongoing "double bind," where a person was damned if she did and damned if she didn't. In a 1956 paper, Bateson and his team explained that a primary injunction or command was verbally delivered to the subject: "Do so and so, or I will punish you" or "Do not do so and so, or I will punish you." Then a more abstract, nonverbal secondary injunction was delivered, which conflicted with the first: "Do not see this as punishment." Finally, a tertiary negative injunction prohibited the subject from escaping the situation. Naturally the person became "excessively concerned with hidden meanings... characteristically suspicious and defiant." This paradigm had echoes of Fromm-Reichmann, whom Bateson et al. cited. But the double bind, as they described it, did not have to involve mothers or even parents. It could result from any human interactions.

There surely was no shortage of "binds" in the Morlok family, and some of these appeared to be compounded by their fame. As investigators could plainly see, the quadruplets were always having to discern what the public expected of them. Sadie's assembled scrapbooks constituted a kind of secondary injunction, making abstract demands of the sisters that conflicted with her and Carl's stated expectations. There was, for instance, immense disparity between parental demands for family secrecy and Sadie's public proclamations that the quadruplets were "everybody's children." While Carl was drawing the blinds and forbidding his daughters even from playing in neighbors' yards, Sadie was telling reporters, "I always adored twins, so I can't blame people for looking at my children."

If investigators were stirred by their observations of the family, they were surely disappointed by the fact that one-on-one sessions with three of the quadruplets were bearing little fruit. Edna, Wilma, and Helen showed no interest in psychotherapy, leaving them to rely on Sarah and the parents' testimonies.

From the beginning, the quadruplets exhibited a combination of resentment and affection for the people who studied and cared for them. Their feelings depended upon the day, the individual in question, and, in Helen's case, the sex. Helen strongly preferred men whenever contact was involved, such as when she was getting her hair washed.

With the exception of Sarah, the quadruplets' conditions also fluctuated, often seeming to correlate with personal disappointments, rather than the nature of the experiments. Shortly after arriving at NIMH, Edna appeared to be doing very well. She'd become friendly with the brother of another patient who visited the ward and had begun to groom herself in preparation for his visits, indicating her potential for eventual independence. She soon found herself vying against Sarah for the man's attention but maintained her spirits. Perhaps she even enjoyed the sibling rivalry, a throwback to their old school days. But then she began to hallucinate and refuse food. Staff often found her in her room weeping. Noting that the suitor had stopped visiting the ward, they presumed romantic disappointments were to blame.

Edna at least had the wherewithal to write her mother for help. She begged Sadie to come, claiming to be under "a mental shock from an experience." Certain that she was pregnant, both Sadie and Carl came at once. One can only wonder what vitriol Carl spewed thinking that his worst fear had come to life. When the Morloks arrived, Edna told her mother that her boyfriend had tried to engage her in sex play. He'd grabbed her breast and "pretended to milk it." Edna further claimed that men were coming into her room with "tension machines" and spoke of "controls" telling her not to bathe.

Edna benefited from her parents' visit but deteriorated even further after they returned to Lansing. She reported suicidal ideations, blurred vision, numbness, and persistent nightmares. She also became convinced someone was holding her down to give her a "death prescription." She heard voices and saw demons with fire around them. Believing they were after Carl, and evidently still feeling responsible for the parent who'd long regarded her as a second wife, she repeatedly proclaimed, "I have to save my father." At one point, she became convinced she and Sarah were going to die in three days. Then she heard God declare that she would be saved from death. She eventually improved only to relapse again a few months later. This was her pattern—up and down, never quite managing to cling onto sanity for very long.

Wilma also wavered, though her psychosis took more aggressive forms. She was very hostile to her parents whenever they were present. When hallucinating, she would scream at the top of her lungs and smash glasses, once even attacking a staff member. She had many compulsions, such as digging through wastebaskets, straightening magazines, cleaning ashtrays, rearranging drawers, and putting her garments in what looked to staff like geometric patterns. Never did she pass through a door without touching both handles. Mostly, though, she would stand in place for prolonged periods of the day.

When her symptoms were more controlled, Wilma cooperated with staff. She'd allow people to dress her and even sought their assistance with other tasks. She would move about the ward and help shelve books in one of the public rooms. She took pains to look attractive, arranging her hair and heavily applying makeup. Staff were pleased to see her effort, even if they thought she looked like a clown.

The person who most wished for Wilma's health, however, was Helen. The youngest Morlok constantly asked about her longtime companion, though she saw her daily even after the quadruplets were assigned new roommates. Sometimes when a staff member was attending to her, Helen would say, "Wilma needs you" or "Give Wilma the pill." Perhaps she thought only one of them could be well and she did not deserve the chance. According to one psychiatrist who treated her, she was convinced of her badness, perpetually expectant of punishment for something, and "always apologizing for living." Perhaps, on the other hand, Helen was simply uninterested in therapeutic regimens for herself. She often refused to go to group sessions or meet with her therapist, claiming to be "very busy." Once in a while, she would ask for her therapist, then claim to be unavailable when he arrived. She giggled about shenanigans like this and the voices, too. In contrast to her sisters, Helen appeared to be amused by her hallucinations, joking with them as she went about her tasks. Her psychosis seemed to provide the friendships that the world had long denied her.

The ward staff came to think of her as a Cinderella figure, even verbally encouraging her for taking initiative to tidy public areas.

Helen often replied to their compliments with a nasty remark, then softened. Though she never seemed to regain a firm grasp of reality while at NIMH, she showed significant improvement when it came to social interaction. She loved to go for long walks with staff and took interest in other patients on the ward, once baking a cake and serving it to them. When told by a physician how special she was, she "glowed." At a Halloween party, this same doctor asked her to dance, and while she declined, he wrote in a patient progress report that he would not be surprised if, in a year, they were doing the bunny hop together. The note marked a rare display of feeling on the page. Most of the sisters' surviving records show clinicians hiding behind medicalese.

When she was in more serious bouts of psychosis, Helen's notions of inadequacy predominated. She would cry, then try to comfort herself, saying "That's all right, dear," in a motherly tone. If her actual mother happened to be visiting, she did not leave her side. Staff knew Helen was in a really bad way when she no longer desired physical contact with male attendants. Or when she began to throw and bang objects such as her dinner tray, warning, "I'm going wild, I'm going wild, I'm going to tip everything over." Sometimes the voices she heard appeared to be sexually provocative. One minute she'd laugh riotously and the next, take on a puritanical voice. In therapy, she sat wordless, though she did deny involvement with the janitor and once offered without provocation, "They burned me, you know."

Because her psychotherapy sessions were unproductive, she was still going without any effective treatment. So were Edna and Wilma. At any other public institution, they'd likely have been administered chlorpromazine. Smith, Kline & French had managed to persuade state hospital administrators that the drug, now in tablet form and going by the brand name Thorazine, would revolutionize asylum care. After some psychiatrists had doubted its efficacy, one dubbing it "psychiatric aspirin" and others expressing concerns of side effects, such as involuntary movements resembling Parkinson's disease, the company had launched a massive marketing campaign, which specifically appealed to psychiatrists' Freudian sensibilities, to get hospital staff to prescribe it. Ads in medical journals claimed that the drug made disturbed patients more receptive to psychotherapy.

Sarah needed no boost to bare her soul. Meeting with Dr. Perlin four times a week for a total of approximately six hundred hours, the third sister was experiencing the kind of therapeutic transformation Rosenthal had witnessed on the battlefield all those years ago. In doing so, she was beginning to carve a life for herself apart from her sisters.

In line with the methods of the day, Perlin's strategy was to fashion himself as a parent figure who listened more than he talked. By recognizing Sarah's suffering without moralizing, and by providing a screen for her to project her feelings for her real father and mother, he intended to help her to make those feelings known to herself. In naming them, she could loosen their grip.

To facilitate her transference, Perlin early on asked Sarah to furnish him with a list titled "Why I Fail to Tell Dr. Perlin Things About Him That Annoy Me." Here she wrote such reasons as "I'm afraid I'll upset him" and "I am afraid I'll lose him as a doctor." She claimed to censor herself depending on the mood or disposition she presumed him to be in. This surely indicated therapeutic progress, as it called to mind the notoriously unstable Carl. Eventually, Sarah managed to make the jump to her father, enumerating why it had been difficult for her to express annoyance with him when living in Lansing. Many of her points were nearly identical to those she'd articulated about Perlin.

In therapy, Sarah also identified her sexual shame, writing that she could more readily accept the fact of sex and "[her]self physically." As she became more comfortable within her own body—her *adult* body—she dated other patients on the ward, allowing some of them to put their arm around her and even kiss her.

Her greatest achievement was learning to view herself both as a quadruplet and a discrete person. "I can have something in common with my sisters or family and still possess my own individuality," she came to believe. Breaking away from the tetrad entailed the greatest psychic risk because it meant confronting the possibility that her sisters might never become well with her. In addition to guilt and a sense of maternal failure (she'd always thought of herself as a surrogate mother), she experienced a kind of terror at having to brave the world alone. She once told Perlin about a dream to this effect. She and Edna were standing in a crowd that resembled the ocean. The waves grew bigger, jostling them. She became very scared, but Edna appeared blithe about the danger they faced. It was like she knew there was an awful wave about to crush them, and she was just going to go down with it. Sarah had to beg and plead with her to get to shore, which they eventually did. Ever since having the dream, Sarah couldn't take a shower without feeling that she was going to be washed away.

Perlin asked what she made of the dream. "As I look at my sisters," she replied, "they just seem so unconcerned, as if nothing ever happened. They just don't care about a thing." And because they'd retreated from the world, they weren't having the terrible time that she was.

Sarah could see how their altered psychological state provided a refuge from reality, where the true terrors lie. With Perlin's help, she was also beginning to grasp how the land of make-believe could become so familiar to a person that she couldn't imagine leaving it behind without losing some integral part of herself. Part of the work of therapy, then, was to answer the question: Who was she without her symptoms?

In early 1957, Sarah took the bold step of leaving the ward to find out. She began to volunteer for NIH's Lab of Nutrition & Endocrinology, which was housed in the same building. Every morning, she'd don her white lab coat, ride the elevator up to the ninth floor, and help with secretarial tasks: reading and recording experiment results, sorting files, and typing two researchers' doctoral theses. The job gave her the sense that she had something to offer and that she really *could* make it on her own. She soon informed her parents that she planned to leave NIMH and take a paid position in DC. As Carl happened to be ill, he did not put up a fight.

After passing a civil service exam, but while still living at the institute, she went to work for the National Naval Medical Center (now Walter Reed National Military Medical Center). There she typed and edited the medical histories of US presidents, active-duty naval officers, marine corps, and other enlisted people. She looked for apartments in the city and took driving lessons. Her very first lesson took her down Pennsylvania Avenue in the middle of a downpour. She'd never forget feeling so scared and thrilled at once.

Like a flower uncurling its petals for the morning sun, she was opening up to the world. After a lifetime of seclusion, she couldn't believe what beauties and mysteries it held. Some wonderful essence enchanted everything, and it seemed to have been there all along. And then one morning while working at the medical center, she got a phone call that changed life as she was beginning to know it. It was her mother on the other end with news that sent her racing back to her sisters in the ward: Carl was dead.

Chapter Eleven

No sooner had NIMH staff learned of Carl's passing than they gathered the quadruplets before a psychiatrist to talk about their feelings. Edna, Wilma, and Helen just sat there with empty stares. Sarah suggested psychoanalysis could wait. "It's time to plan the trip home," she said. "We have to get our things together and get ready for takeoff." She then coordinated with a nurse to book air travel and choose mourning clothes for her sisters.

One sociologist and two nurses traveled with them to Lansing for Carl's funeral, which occurred on the Monday following his death. When she saw her father's casket, Edna broke down in tears. Wilma grew very angry, and Helen appeared not to register the events. Only Sarah was able to greet guests alongside her mother, later staying behind to help write thank-you cards to all who attended the ceremony or sent flowers. She felt remorseful for not having been there when Carl became sick, even though Sadie had told her not to come, saying he would be insufferable.

Indeed, after his hospital admission for cirrhosis of the liver, Carl was defiant as ever. He'd barked at all the nurses and once rolled toilet paper all the way down the hall, past their station, and then back again. He later tried to choke his wife, having to be restrained in a straitjacket. It was as if he knew death was about to level him and refused to go quietly so as never to be remembered as anything but a strong man, a man who was in charge.

The *State Journal* had only praise for Carl, eulogizing him as "a conscientious public official of splendid reputation." The newspaper made no mention of the scientific studies under way, even though staff were presumably aware—an editor had honored David Rosenthal and Olive Quinn's request for copies of all stories on the family.

Once back at NIMH, Edna, Wilma, and Helen grew more disturbed. Edna turned silent, disappointing staff members who thought she'd recently turned a corner. Wilma and Helen began to act out. Sarah admitted she was depressed but managed not to lose her bearings.

Investigators took interest in their mourning, though probably not nearly as much as they would have if they'd been more attuned to figures like the Hungarian psychoanalyst Sándor Ferenczi and Austrian British psychoanalyst Anna Freud (Sigmund's daughter). Ferenczi believed sexual trauma underlay far more pathologies than was acknowledged and that many children identified with those who'd harmed them. In a 1932 conference paper, later revised and published in the *International Journal of Psychoanalysis*, he theorized this was because trauma robbed children of their senses, putting them into a dissociative trance wherein they became transfixed by the desires and behaviors of their aggressor. In his words, children were easily disoriented by a "confusion of tongues," whereby abusers didn't just threaten and scare, but provided affection and security. Anna Freud expounded upon the notion of "identification with the aggressor." In a 1936 book chapter, which neither named Ferenczi nor focused on sexual abuse, she suggested that such identification was a defense mechanism intended to protect the self from hurt and disorganization. By taking on the identity of the person who had harmed them, a child felt empowered.

It stands to reason that it would've been even easier for the quadruplets to identify with—and then mourn—their abusive father, given how the press lionized Carl and named society's outsiders as the true menace. But the quadruplets' identification with their father was not really under scrutiny, as many investigators did not appear to view abuse as having driven them mad. Whereas Ferenczi or Freud might have thought their collective disorder a form of reminiscence—every tic and grimace pointing back to Carl or some other perpetrator—the family-minded researchers remained more focused on the sisters' identification with Sadie, which they believed had inhibited them from forming self-concepts. This was despite the fact that many sympathized with Sadie because of her own abuse at Carl's hands. According to Rosenthal and two colleagues, "When her husband died, the expressions of sympathy that she received were not so much concerned with her bereavement but with all that she had to bear before his death." This outpouring stood in sharp contrast to that of Sadie's friends and relatives back home.

Not long after Carl's death, Sarah took the step of leaving the Clinical Center for a full-time job. She'd made much progress in psychotherapy, coming to understand certain truths about herself, such as her desperate need to please others. She decided she would continue to meet with Dr. Perlin, but not other support staff. That way, she would have someone to help her work through any conflicts that arose while maintaining some independence.

Life on the outside did not go as hoped. As she told Perlin, a woman at the job "dominated" her, and she began to have fantasies of being swallowed whole by this person. Frightened, she quit and returned to NIMH. It wasn't the first and it wouldn't be the last moment in her life when she thought she'd made it, only to feel her otherness.

It's hard to tell if Sarah was singled out for abuse or if she merely couldn't cope as well as her peers in the midcentury workplace, where women often resorted to bullying one another as a way of proving their worth to men. All her life, Sarah *had* been an object of scorn, often because others perceived her and her sisters to be strange and vulnerable. At the same time, she was unusually sensitive to criticism, interpreting any shortcoming as a barrier to friendship. In her words, "Being perfect [was her] way of getting closer to people."

Shortly after being readmitted to NIMH, she received news that Perlin was leaving to be married. She was devastated, as she'd actually fallen in love with him. She had once confessed this in a session. Though it was common for patients to develop feelings for their therapist, he appeared taken aback. According to her, "He had a rather angry look on his face but didn't say anything."

Without Perlin, Sarah didn't see any reason to stay at the Clinical Center. She again began to make plans to leave, this time with a social worker to facilitate her transition. The two of them agreed that she should try Woodley House, a soon-to-open psychiatric halfway house in the city. Conceived by an occupational therapist at the nearby St. Elizabeths Hospital, Woodley House was designed for people whose distress was not severe enough to require intensive treatment but who needed support returning to the community. It was all the better that the staff at the home neither asked for nor intended to keep case histories of residents. Patients were admitted on the basis of two questions, to be answered by their therapist: What was the worst thing that might happen to the patient, and what was the best? This meant Sarah could have a fresh start. No one needed to know anything about her family except what she chose to reveal.

It wasn't only Sarah who was leaving NIMH. As 1957 drew to a close, Sadie decided the time had come for all her daughters to move on. Edna, Wilma, and Helen were really no better than when they'd first been admitted. If Sadie was bitter about this fact, she didn't say so, only making arrangements for her more troubled daughters to transfer to Northville State Hospital in Detroit, where they were sure to be put on a pill regimen. The FDA had now approved various derivatives of chlorpromazine, whose effects were proclaimed to be just as miraculous as those of Thorazine.

In the new year, Sarah moved into Woodley House, while the others returned to Michigan. Never again would all four live under the same roof. Sarah found her new domicile to be "a home-like and cozy place," raving to her new housemates and staff members about the fireplace, the beautiful French doors, and the friendly people. Feeling warmth around her, she shared her struggles with being "one-quarter of a person" and her excitement about this new chapter in her life. She had no idea her affection wasn't immediately reciprocated.

The diary of Joan Doniger, the founder of Woodley House, which was eventually turned over to NIMH investigators, offers insight into the disdain for her. "She is a gusher," wrote Doniger. "She sounds enthusiastic about coming, and I will like having her. But I'm apprehensive. I'm afraid that people will not like her... As an unsophisticated non-intellectual girl, she may not fit with our group, and her gushiness, I admit, is quite embarrassing to me." In another entry, Doniger expressed annoyance with Sarah's overuse of the words *nice*, *lovely*, and *wonderful*. Noting that she used such adjectives to describe everything from the building to the pancakes served at breakfast, she wrote, "It's almost impossible to know what she's really thinking."

Once more, Sarah's impulse to embody sweetness was off-putting.

Would she ever learn to be more authentic, or at least appear so when her effusive feelings were genuine? And if she didn't, would there be anyone to embrace her anyway? What happened to girls who learned to please before they could speak, but who couldn't very well discern what others wanted?

Another staff member objected to another of Sarah's mannerisms. "I don't like her closeness, her touching, her patting," this woman wrote in her own diary. "She makes me uncomfortable." Sarah's psychomotor movements also got under the skin. "She makes a rhythmic motion with her fork. She moves it back and forth and up and down a few times before putting food on it and the fork in her mouth. She did the same thing with her glass."

Perhaps Sarah's perceived awkwardness owed as much to the class disparity between her and her supervisors as to her anxious mental state. Here was a girl from middle America—one raised on homemade dresses and public charity—come face-to-face with two cosmopolitan easterners. Like many a hopeful arriviste before her, Sarah simply didn't know the norms of polite society, which prescribed what was a proper display of feeling and what was boorishly sentimental.

As time went on, however, her idealism endeared her to staff and housemates alike. Everyone could see that she had nerve and courage, taking her health more seriously than most. What was not to admire about someone with such a relentless desire to lead a full life, one not defined by her past? They also noted that Sarah refused to be sucked into feuds among the residents. Whereas others would take sides, she remained impartial, just going about her business. It wasn't until an elderly woman named Bernice came along that anyone saw her get out of sorts.

As Sarah told her social worker, she initially didn't mind the sixty-something-year-old who became her roommate. But then

Bernice began to talk about what an awful place Woodley House was. She went on and on about how ill managed it was and how the residents were all being neglected. Sarah became afraid all the negativity was going to make her relapse. She feared discord like the plague, leading her social worker to understand that her positivity was as much for her own mental health as for anyone else. One day she finally snapped. Bernice was pestering another resident with a series of personal questions, and she interrupted, "Mind your own business!" Another time, Bernice put on a dress and complained that it made her look like a horse. "Yes, it does," said a smug Sarah. She knew it wasn't kind, but she couldn't help herself.

Many staff members grew concerned when Sarah took a job in the city and then began to work overtime. Sometimes she didn't come home until seven thirty, eating a cold supper in the kitchen. It didn't help that she'd also begun to date, often choosing to go on romantic outings instead of joining the group for picnics or other events. Even though the whole idea behind Woodley House was helping people reintegrate into society, some feared she was moving too quickly.

One of Sarah's chores was to do the dishes, and a woman named Mary often kept her company, listening as she talked about men she was dating and one crush at Woodley House. Sarah once confided that a boyfriend had kissed her good night without permission. The incident had made her very upset, and she wanted to know if Mary had ever had such an experience. Another time, she said a total stranger had picked her up off the ground during her lunch hour. She'd already told her social worker about it but couldn't shake the bad feelings.

"Some things that happen are not reflections of ourselves," Mary offered. "If someone tried to pick you up, it doesn't mean it's your fault or that you are to blame." It was the first time Sarah had ever heard such words, and she let Mary know how helpful they were.

The younger women at Woodley House shared many secrets as they ironed, hemmed, and did one another's hair. These hours together were some of Sarah's most blissful, as they reminded her of the days when Wilma had set up her beauty shop in the family home. Sometimes, when they'd been lucky, Carl had stayed out of their way long enough for them to forget they had nowhere to go all gussied up. It was one of the small, stolen joys that had helped them to survive.

After a year, Sarah grew lonesome for her real sisters. As Christmas approached, she made plans to return to Lansing to see her family. On her way to the airport, someone stopped her with a box of cookies. Mary caught the surprise and pleasure in her eyes, later musing that even after all this time, Sarah couldn't quite believe people cared about her. Upon returning, she was a basket case. All anyone could coax out of her was that her sisters were in bad shape.

According to hospital notes later acquired by NIMH, Edna's grasp of reality had improved since her admission to the state hospital, but her affect and behavior had not. She wore a fixed smile, made constant sucking noises through her teeth, and just stared into space. She had resigned herself to the idea of hospitalization, viewing it as inevitable. If asked why she was there, she replied, "Mother thinks we need more supervision." Pressed to explain why, she replied, "Well, multiple births are a more nervous temperament." In what way? "Well, we're nervous, Mother says." Also concerning to staff was her involvement with a patient named Lenny. Edna often disappeared with this man for a few hours at a time, sending attendants into a tizzy as they searched the ward for them. Once while watching a movie with other patients, she began to fumble with his clothes. Her lack of inhibition was troubling, but as far as staff knew, Edna's sex play never progressed beyond petting.

Wilma was still hearing voices, now those of her mother and close friends telling her what to do. Her speech was incoherent, and staff had to probe for her thoughts, as she often claimed to be too troubled to discuss them. She'd picked up smoking and would grow very irritated if running low on cigarettes. (Sadie always brought them when she visited.) At least she still had her sense of humor, and would imitate television personalities. She had become involved in group activities, and she often contributed poems to the hospital magazine and volunteered at the in-house beauty shop. Her boss there thought she had talent and suggested she go to cosmetology school, but the doctors didn't think she was well enough.

Helen was the most withdrawn, sometimes refusing to speak with staff. She loathed being watched or told what to do and would often swear under her breath. She frequently urinated in bed and admitted to hearing words, though she denied voices. To her credit, she generally complied with ward rules and even took comfort in some routines. She loved to watch cartoons in the lounge and could often be heard cackling at the happenings on-screen.

The drugs that were now flooding the market had not cured any of them. Edna had started on Thorazine, then switched to Trilafon. Wilma was on Thorazine, and Helen was taking Stelazine and Compazine. Though these antipsychotics had varying mechanisms of action, they all appeared to arrest the nervous system, leading some skeptics to denounce the new class of drugs as psychiatry's latest means to control patients. NIMH psychiatrist Lawrence Kolb called Thorazine "physically more harmful than morphine and heroin." It wouldn't be long before others found that, while the drugs did appear to reduce psychotic episodes, they did nothing to remedy the so-called negative symptoms of schizophrenia, including flat affect, apathy, and inability to experience pleasure. Still others would claim that antipsychotics had the potential to *produce* psychosis in people with schizophrenia, a prospect that surely would have troubled the Morloks.

But the drug industry was getting the better of its critics, leaving no question as to the direction of Edna, Wilma, and Helen's treatment. Enthralled by the idea of a miracle pill, reporters now satirized "ivory-tower psychoanalysts" who refused to endorse the new therapy. In the words of one *TIME* magazine contributor, such holdouts were still trying to figure out if their patient "withdrew from the world because of unconscious conflict over incestuous urges or stealing from his brother's piggy bank at the age of five." To the "red-brick pragmatists" (those working in public hospitals), this was like "arguing about the number of angels on the head of a pin." It was precisely such caricatures that inclined many psychiatrists to get behind the new drugs. In the likes of Thorazine, "mind doctors" saw an opportunity to be taken as seriously as other practitioners of medicine. Even in the very recent heyday of talk therapy, they'd never been as esteemed as surgeons and cardiologists. Here was their chance.

After seeing Edna, Wilma, and Helen in such bad shape, Sarah became even more determined to put her own psychiatric treatment behind her. It seems that seeing the light gone out of them made her adamant to keep her own burning. In January, she began to make plans to leave Woodley House. Her social worker was apprehensive, suggesting she first have a trial visit away, but Sarah insisted she was ready. In that case, her social worker responded, she should know that she would always be welcome back. With this reassurance, Sarah moved into a YWCA home in the city. Once there, she found a new job that didn't require overtime and became involved at Luther Place Memorial Lutheran Church.

Luther Place was an evangelical Lutheran church like the one she'd attended in Lansing. But it was part of the mainline tradition, not a theologically conservative synod. Its founding pastor, the Reverend John Butler, had been an abolitionist who believed Christians' purpose on earth was to bind wounds, not inflict them. In accordance with this mission, Luther Place based its ministry in social justice and community-building. Church came to have new meaning for the woman who hadn't even been permitted to socialize after her confirmation lessons. It was no longer a place where she went simply to learn the "right" beliefs, but one where she got to break bread with people who dreamed of peace and harmony on earth.

It was in such a circle of dreamers that she fell in love. She'd never forget the first moment she saw George Cotton. She was in a coffee line after Sunday service, and a woman was introducing her to all the people there. A tall and handsome man in military uniform was watching her as she made her way down the line to him. When she got to shaking his hand, she could sense his interest. They began chatting about different committees to volunteer on. She mentioned an interest in the choir, and so it wasn't any surprise when he joined, too.

One night after a rehearsal, everyone in the choir went out to dinner. She happened to be seated next to another man, and George came up and muttered an excuse as to why he should sit next to her. They nervously exchanged pleasantries, and then he worked up the courage to ask her on a date. He didn't care that she was six years older than him.

"It was a really happy time in my life," she later wrote of their courtship. He took her to different places around the city, and they became involved with Young People, an organization for young adults at Luther Place. He always wanted to be with her. Once when they were scheduled to go out, he called to say his car battery had died. She told him not to worry and just stay at home. But not long afterward, the clerk in the lobby of her building buzzed to say he was there. He'd hitchhiked.

As was inevitable, she discovered certain flaws. George was frivolous with money and rather fond of drinking. These traits bothered her enough to briefly end things and date a police officer before going back to him. In October 1959, some months before he was to deploy for Saudi Arabia, he asked her to marry him. He'd bought a ring at Bolling Air Force Base, where he was stationed. She felt more ambivalent about the proposal than she imagined she would. Her feet grew colder when he refused to go to Lansing to meet her family over the Christmas holiday. He said he had other plans and, besides, it was only her he was marrying.

That spring, when she still hadn't committed one way or the other, he urged her to meet with an air force chaplain. Girlfriends couldn't live on base, this man pointed out. And the military didn't really look out for girlfriends, only real wives. If she wanted to have a future with George, she had to tie the knot.

Just like her mother before her, Sarah acquiesced to the pressure. Perhaps wanting some semblance of control, she declared that she wanted to get married in Lansing. That way, her sisters could be in the wedding. Both Edna and Wilma were now out of the state hospital. Edna was living with their mother, who had taken in boarders for income. She had a job and small circle of friends. She'd tried to kindle a romance with Lenny, the fellow from the hospital, paying him to come visit her at home. Sadie had disapproved of the arrangement—not because it involved cash but because she thought the guy lazy. Though she claimed no current interest in dating or marriage, Edna was irate to learn about Sarah's engagement. So was Wilma, who pouted to their mother, "There should have been a quadruplet wedding!"

Now living in a halfway house and attending beauty school in Detroit, Wilma's own romantic hopes had also been dashed. While in the hospital, she'd begun to date a patient named Thomas. Nervous that she was overinvested in the relationship, hospital staff had assigned him to another ward. This sent her back into a catatonic state. She spent hours frozen in place and refused to eat. Likely because of her weight loss, she did not menstruate for five months. Just to be sure she hadn't broken her pose and gone to find her lover, staff sent her for a pregnancy test, which came back negative.

Thomas was actually an ex-boyfriend of Helen, who gave no indication of being ready for discharge. The youngest Morlok had dated the man after gaining work and roaming privileges at the hospital, which boasted a gymnasium, movie theater, swimming pool, and bowling alley. The two conspired to meet at different locations on the grounds, often not returning to the ward when they were supposed to. Citing sexual acting-out on Helen's part, the staff revoked her privileges, at which point Thomas turned to Wilma. He once wrote a letter to Helen professing his preference for her. Only after this did Helen regress and become mute. Never in her life had she been anyone's favorite, and others had gone and sabotaged it. When she finally recovered her voice, she began to excessively apply makeup and was friendlier than ever before. According to her sisters, she always thought her sexuality her greatest asset. Her daringness really peeved Wilma, who once told their mother, "Men only prefer Helen because she will do things that I won't do."

Helen was the only sister who wasn't bothered by Sarah's

engagement. "That's nice," she said upon hearing the news. But she was not deemed well enough to attend the ceremony, which ultimately took place in Ohio, where George's parents lived. Only Sadie and Edna attended, Edna serving as maid of honor.

Sarah wore a white ballerina gown of soft white satin, a seed pearl veil, and a gold-plated crucifix gifted by her groom. Before the ceremony, her mother, fashionably attired in a navy dress and matching straw hat, took her aside, looked her deep in the eyes, and wished her love, peace, and happiness. It was a tender moment that Carl undoubtedly would have tried to spoil—if he'd even agreed to be present for this momentous occasion in his daughter's life. But he was gone now, and even the deepest wounds had begun to heal. After decades of estrangement, Sadie had also made good with her siblings, one of whom gave Sarah away. Another had previously taken in Wilma, though Wilma's excessive smoking had doomed the arrangement.

The day after the wedding, a few friends drove Sarah and her new husband back to Washington, where they found an apartment to last them until George deployed for the Middle East. Then Sarah was off to live with her in-laws, working for a nationally known aviation company where her father-in-law was employed. Monday through Friday, she would get up, scarf down a banana, and drive the two of them to the office. In the evenings and on weekends, she chauffeured her mother-in-law around town and ran errands for her.

Eventually, she grew to dislike the woman, finding her jealous and abusive. She did not understand why she had to be the elder Mrs. Cotton's servant when she paid for room and board. She also resented that her in-laws mocked her for wanting to go to church. One day Sarah's mother-in-law caught her husband in bed with another woman. If he was sleeping around, she reasoned, he must be going behind her back with Sarah. Enraged, she moved all of Sarah's belongings to the garage. Sarah called her mother and begged to be rescued. Sadie listened calmly and then promptly arranged for a moving truck to transport her stuff to Lansing, where she stayed until George was transferred to a base in England.

As Sarah prepared to join him there, Sadie expressed some misgivings about the marriage, mostly relating to George's drinking and selfishness—the very qualities that likened him to Carl. Her caution was soon forgotten, as Sarah's next few years were some of her most jubilant. She and her husband spent weekends climbing the Tower of London and wandering the perimeter of Buckingham Palace. Riding double-decker buses around the city and getting their pictures taken with the famous Beefeater guards. Driving up to Scotland to marvel at the shaggy-haired Highland cattle and then looking in the dark waters for the Loch Ness monster.

With George working on base, Sarah took a clerical position at a law firm. The money was so good she didn't even mind sitting in the back so no one knew an American worked there. She loved going to court and seeing the barristers in their wigs of white curls. They all spoke so eloquently until the bells rang for teatime and everyone stopped what they were doing to drink and take crumpets. It delighted her that the whole city came together for this routine.

Society was not so rosy stateside. The US was entering one of the most tumultuous decades of the century, as civil rights activists took to the streets and were met with bullets, police batons, fire hoses, and armored tanks. The Cold War between the US and Soviet Union raged on, providing a pretext for J. Edgar Hoover and other federal authorities to erode civil liberties and stoke such paranoia that many regarded their neighbors and co-workers with deep suspicion. The conflict in Vietnam was also escalating, with

Americans fearing US involvement. Despite all this, many had a sense of hope. The Reverend Dr. King was leading Black Americans ever closer to the promised land, and President Kennedy had a plan to send Americans to the moon, as well as to establish equal pay for women and fair labor standards for all workers. As the music of Camelot played on, Kennedy vowed to fight another social abuse: the disgraceful treatment of the mentally ill.

In October 1963, Kennedy signed into law what became known as the Community Mental Health Act, which allocated millions in federal funding for the development of community mental health centers in the United States. In a speech about the measure, the president proclaimed that "the mentally ill and the mentally retarded need no longer be alien to our affections or beyond the help of our communities." By this, he meant that no longer should the afflicted be warehoused in asylums, where so many horrific practices had taken place. (Undoubtedly, Kennedy was thinking of his own sister Rosemary, whose intellectual disability another sibling had disclosed to the public the previous year.) New drug treatments made it possible for most in state institutions to be returned to their rightful place in society. To close the door on such a shameful chapter of history, Kennedy had also prevailed upon Congress to allocate funding for research on the "harsh environmental conditions" correlated with mental illness, which were then known to include poverty, class inequality, racial inequality, violence, and poor education.

The bill—in fact, the last major one that Kennedy signed before his assassination the following month—marked a victory for the social psychiatry espoused by NIMH director Robert Felix, as it essentially authorized the federal government to bypass the states and become involved in the mental health of the nation like never before. But it was arguably a far greater boon for biological psychiatry, as it signaled a shift away from psychoanalytic principles toward prescription drugs. It was amid this turning of the tide—from Freud to "pharma"—that David Rosenthal published his edited volume on the Morlok sisters, suggesting a genetic basis of schizophrenia. The book excited scientific circles, with some experts understanding Rosenthal to have amicably resolved the nature-nurture debate, even though he emphasized it was only a single case study. Perhaps some were influenced by the hope that pills would prove to be the panacea that experts were claiming. It stood to reason that a condition with biological origins could be ameliorated by biological treatments.

But it remained to be seen what, if anything, either genetics research or drugs would do for the quadruplets or the millions of others with serious mental illness, who were soon to find far less community support than Kennedy promised. For reasons having much to do with the unrest in the streets, public attitudes about schizophrenia and other social crises were about to transform in ways that neither the president nor other proponents of the Community Mental Health Act could possibly have imagined.

Chapter Twelve

When the Reverend Dr. Martin Luther King, Jr., first rose to prominence following the 1955 Montgomery bus boycott, David Rosenthal was one of the many white Americans to regard him skeptically. The Alabama preacher claimed nonviolent methods, but the media portrayed him as vengeful.

As the civil rights movement gained steam, many of Rosenthal's peers began to describe activists as split between desiring peace and revenge—in a word, schizophrenic. King himself used the term to denote the pull toward good and evil, or violence and nonviolence. But for psychiatrists like Walter Bromberg and Franck Simon, the connection between Black liberation and schizophrenia was not metaphorical; the crusade for equality *literally* caused delusions, hallucinations, and violent projections in Black men. On the basis of such logic, the FBI diagnosed activist Malcolm X as having pre-psychotic paranoid schizophrenia. Never mind that the government was profiling and tapping his phone; his fear of the state was totally beyond the pale. His mother had also been an agitator with delusions about white people. Her name: Louise Little. After spending twenty-four years in Kalamazoo State Hospital, the object of Lansing welfare officials' disdain was finally released in 1963. The state would later send the family a petition for reimbursement for her "care" in the amount of $13,000 (about $24,000 today).

According to psychiatrist Jonathan Metzl, pharmaceutical companies swiftly tapped into the pervasive racial anxiety, which resurfaced slavery-era notions of pathological mischief-making on the part of freedom seekers. Drug advertisements in medical journals began to portray maniacal Black men alongside promises of psychotropics' calming effects. "Assaultive and belligerent?" asked one such ad, showing a man with clenched fist and mouth wide open. "Cooperation often begins with Haldol." At a time when white Americans were resorting to all manner of violence to protect the racial hierarchy, Big Pharma was touting its own solution: chemical incarceration.

Rosenthal did not lend his voice to this recoding of schizophrenia as a Black disease, which would soon pollute NIMH studies and even the second edition of the *Diagnostic and Statistical Manual.* Despite the racist caricatures coming from within his profession, and despite the considerable effort on the part of the press and the FBI to present King as a grave threat to white Americans, Rosenthal became convinced it was a sincere champion of peace whose face so often came on his television screen. Perhaps because he'd endured discrimination himself, he supported the civil rights movement, the effects of which would soon reverberate in his personal life. He further kept focused on the study of schizophrenia's transmission through both genetics and familial environment.

Nevertheless his 1963 book on the schizophrenic quadruplets fueled a public research agenda that located pathology in the person and that posited pills, not hours of talk therapy, as the solution. Despite containing only one chapter from the perspective of a geneticist and many more from the psychologists, sociologists, and social workers who'd analyzed the family, the fate of *The Genain Quadruplets* was already written.

In a theoretical overview concluding the massive volume, Rosenthal proposed that some inherited factor provided a constitutional host for the sisters' mental illness, without which "Nora," "Iris," "Myra," and "Hester" would never have gone mad. (Following the lead of Dr. Haynes's daughter, Rosenthal drew upon the letters N-I-M-H.) In support of this theory, he noted the "widespread psychiatric disorders in the paternal family" and the quadruplets' own exhibition of schizophrenic personality traits from a very early age: "They had low energy levels, were rather placid, 'sweet,' introversive, not very talkative." His chosen pseudonym for the family placed further emphasis on biology's primordial role. *Genain* came from the Greek words for "dire birth," or "dreadful gene."

But that wasn't the end of the story. The quadruplets' misfortune was "an unhappy collusion of nature and nurture." Citing Paul Meehl's model of "diathesis-stress," wherein schizophrenic disorder emerged when a person with some predisposition was exposed to stress, Rosenthal described their home environment as being thoroughly pathogenic. Both parents "practiced" irrationality, and there were both vertical and horizontal identification patterns within the family, meaning that the quadruplets over-identified with their parents and each other. They tended to echo their mother's words, sometimes in a chain. Edna, especially, gave the impression that she had "no single thought, no mental life, no repertoire of verbal response that she [could] call her own."

It wasn't just that familial dysfunction *manifested* psychosis; it also seemed to have shaped the sisters' respective courses of illness. Building on the work of his colleague Lyman Wynne, Rosenthal noted that outsiders could not distinguish the sisters' personalities when they were young and differences in parental treatment were presumably less pronounced. All were said to be shy and withdrawn. Only over the years, as their parents selected discrete roles for each of them, did their behavioral tendencies harden into those now on display. This was not to say that their personalities were entirely socially constructed—it was probably innate propensities that had influenced their parents' casting choices. But the sisters' defining characteristics clearly coordinated with parental expectations of them, which were then extended to the school setting. After years of being favored, Sarah and Edna had the better prognoses, while the disfavored daughters, Wilma and Helen, were in worse shape.

Curiously, Rosenthal also gestured toward psychologist Bruno Bettelheim's "extreme situation." In a 1943 paper reflecting on his experiences in German concentration camps, Bettelheim had argued that terrorized individuals rationally adapted to their circumstances with psychic disintegration—a process that was uncannily similar to the development of schizophrenia in children. In Rosenthal's words, the quadruplets were "overpowered... in constant jeopardy [and unable to] protect themselves." Their mother surely smothered them, but it was their father who was the greatest menace. As they could not predict his rages, they were always waiting for the other shoe to drop. The outside world "provided no truly comforting respite." Both at school and onstage, they endured taunts and abuse.

With these few remarks, Rosenthal put pressure on those of his contributors who were narrowly focused on the schizophrenogenic mother, in addition to suggesting that the quadruplets' wider milieu had been corrosive.

Despite the intrigue of comparing the quadruplets to Holocaust victims, and despite his "remarkable balance," to quote one reviewer, it was his discussion of genetic vulnerability that principally occupied medical-scientific audiences when he traveled the country to speak about the quadruplets. The possibility of separating the effects of nature and nurture also absorbed his peers. In the quadruplets' case, it had been impossible to segment the two, but many researchers, including his colleague and contributor Seymour Kety, still believed it could be done.

So did Leonard Heston, an Oregon psychiatrist who set out to compare children born to schizophrenic mothers and then given up for adoption with adopted children whose biological mother was not schizophrenic. In 1966, Heston published a study reporting that five of his forty-seven index adoptees had traits associated with schizophrenia, while none of the control adoptees did. Though he admitted to being involved in both the psychiatric interviews and diagnostic process (not exactly meeting the standards of a blind review), and though he never specified his diagnostic criteria, simply claiming to use "generally accepted standards," he had reached the threshold of statistical significance. Had there been one control adoptee found schizophrenic, or one less index adoptee found schizophrenic, the findings would not have reached said threshold.

Kety conceived of another approach to separate nature and nurture. Rather than starting with schizophrenic mothers and examining their given-away children, investigators could look at families of schizophrenics known to have been given up for adoption in infancy or early childhood. If genetics predisposed a person to mental illness, these schizophrenics would have greater incidence of biological family members with schizophrenia than the general population.

Kety organized expansive studies of adoptees in Copenhagen, Denmark, where, at the height of the eugenics era, the government had constructed elaborate national population databases. He asked

Rosenthal to join him for this project, along with a psychiatrist named Paul Wender, who worked at St. Elizabeths, which would come under NIMH's administrative control in 1967. Rosenthal did so, following a six-month stay in Jerusalem, where he had actually delved deeper into environmental stressors by studying the outcomes of children born of schizophrenic parents and reared either by their biological parents or in a communal setting known as a kibbutz. Rosenthal's research in Israel, which found a greater rate of schizophrenic diagnosis in kibbutz-reared children, would never attract the same degree of attention as *The Genain Quadruplets* or the adoption studies he was now embarking upon with Kety.

Kety, Rosenthal, Wender, and a team of Danish and American researchers started by identifying all the individuals born in Copenhagen between the years 1924 and 1947 and given up for adoption at birth or early childhood. From this group of 5,483, they identified 507 people who had been admitted to a psychiatric hospital for any reason and secured those persons' medical records. Three clinicians reviewed the medical records and scored the individuals for definite or possible cases of schizophrenia. There were thirty-three patients whom all three physicians agreed were schizophrenic. The researchers then hunted for mental illness among these schizophrenics' 463 biological and adoptive relatives by searching the Psychiatric Register of the Institute of Human Genetics, the admissions data of fourteen major psychiatric hospitals, police records, military records, and charity records.

Much to the primary investigators' surprise, not one of the identified relatives met the criteria to be marked schizophrenic, though many appeared to suffer from milder conditions, eccentricities, or "inadequate personality," a catchall term that the *DSM* provided for traits like social ineptitude. In response to this finding, Kety and his associates suggested that milder disorders could constitute borderline (or latent) schizophrenia, there being "a schizophrenia spectrum of disorders." By broadening the diagnostic framework, they identified 13 cases among the 150 biological relatives of the index group compared with only 3 cases among the 156 biological relatives of the control group. This was statistically significant, though it left the researchers hard-pressed to explain another finding: More than half of the relatives assigned to the spectrum were not parents or full siblings, but half siblings on the paternal side. The researchers could not account for this but noted that the finding meant that the schizophrenics and their half siblings on the spectrum had shared no environment, not even in utero. They concluded that roughly 10 percent prevalence of the disorder found in the families of naturally reared schizophrenics was a manifestation of genetically transmitted factors.

The researchers also utilized the Danish population databases to expand upon Heston's experiment. In a separate study, this one led by Rosenthal, they considered thirty-nine high-risk, adopted-away offspring of a parent with confirmed schizophrenia, whose adoptive family had no known schizophrenia, then compared the cohort with a control sample of forty-seven adoptees with no schizophrenic biological parents. Looking only at the subjects' history of psychiatric hospitalization, they initially found a statistically insignificant difference between the index and control groups: Only one adoptee in the index group had been hospitalized for schizophrenia, compared with zero in the control. But when they conducted their own evaluation of subjects and utilized their spectrum, they found thirteen positive cases in the index group and seven positive cases in the control group. The rate of disorder in the index group was then more than two times that of the control group—a result that was statistically meaningful.

Kety and Rosenthal first introduced their findings in 1967 at an international conference on "The Transmission of Schizophrenia," which brought together world-renowned epidemiologists, neurophysiologists, genealogists, geneticists, sociologists, and linguists in Dorado Beach, Puerto Rico. Only the year before, Rosenthal had accepted a promotion to chief of the psychology laboratory, following Shakow's retirement. There really had been no question as to who should replace Shakow, though Rosenthal had to be pressured to take the job. "He really didn't enjoy [supervisory] work," his colleague and neighbor Morris Parloff later recalled. "He was basically a very shy man." Rosenthal only agreed on the condition that Parloff help him with some of the routine administration, which would allow him to focus on his research.

According to Carlos Sluzki, a psychoanalyst and family therapist present at the Puerto Rico conference, "the ground trembled" when Rosenthal related that roughly 10 percent of the prevalence of schizophrenia found in non-adoptive families was due to genetically transmitted factors. In Sluzki's summary, "Schizophrenia manifested itself, apparently, on the basis of a genetic load. Nurture appeared to have lost the battle." As in the case of his book, Rosenthal was not quite so partisan, taking care to stress the need for further research into how exactly external stressors brought about illness in persons believed to have genetic predisposition. On the last day of the conference, he even acknowledged the contributions of the nurture camp when he praised all attendees for their open-mindedness: "This week we have been able to sit here day after day and listen to people expounding ideas both compatible and contrary to our own, and far from catching any dread affliction, the only thing we have caught, I hope, is the spirit of earnest concern about the other man's data and opinions." But as Sluzki could see, he and his team had clearly enshrined the study of genetics in psychiatric illness. There really was no going back to the days when the mind sciences largely scorned biological investigations as a matter of course, nor when family studies dominated the research agenda of organizations like the NIMH.

If this elated the biologists, it perturbed psychotherapists like Theodore Lidz, who noted that Kety and Rosenthal had not bothered to examine the family milieu into which children were adopted—they'd simply declared it functional. Lidz also criticized the invention of an elastic spectrum of complaints. "It must be somewhat difficult to know just who should be categorized as a *definite* latent schizophrenic," Lidz wrote in a 1976 paper. But that researchers felt they knew "how to judge with any certainty who may or may not be an *uncertain* latent schizophrenic is a rather extraordinary feat."

Lidz was part of a small but growing movement to become known as anti-psychiatry, many of whose members criticized the re-biologizing of psychiatry on the basis that sanity and madness were philosophical matters, not medical ones. The mind, after all, was not an anatomical organ, but a conglomeration of intangible thoughts, memories, imaginings, desires, fears, beliefs, and emotions. While this view inclined Lidz to regard schizophrenia as a personality disorder, rather than a biological disease, he never actually disputed Kety and Rosenthal's notion that genetics predisposed certain people to become schizophrenic, nor the notion that drugs might be useful in treating certain physical symptoms associated with the disorder. He simply didn't think the question of heredity to be germane. Individuals couldn't very well change their or their children's genetic makeup. They could, however, benefit from healthy interpersonal and family relations learned in therapy.

Other so-called anti-psychiatrists, both in America and around the world, were beginning to push beyond the family and implicate society in the development of disorders like schizophrenia.

According to psychoanalyst R. D. Laing and anthropologist Jules Henry, the dysfunctional family was but a microcosm of a deeply sick and violent world; and mental and emotional disturbances occurred when individuals either resisted or broke down under the abuse. But with many certain they were edging closer to the precise genetic bases of schizophrenia—and with many hankering to pathologize the Black body—few within the establishment were willing to entertain such critiques.

The resistance to considering societal dysfunction may be best captured by the revisions to the *DSM-II*, published in 1968. In the discussion of schizophrenia, experts removed the word *reaction* and recast the paranoid type so that it read less as the malady of a passive, gender-neutral person and more as the malady of the man who posed a threat to the social order. By essentially bidding farewell to the stressed-out heroine of *The Snake Pit* and hello to the likes of Malcolm X, the *DSM* transformed the schizophrenic from a victim to a menace. In this way, the manual utterly failed to meet the supposed standards of that edition: correcting the US-centrism of the first edition. In Metzl's summary, "A diagnostic text meant to shift focus away from the specifics of culture instead became inexorably intertwined with the cultural politics, and above all the race politics, of a particular nation and a particular moment in time."

There were some NIMH researchers, such as Lyman Wynne and Loren Mosher, who continued to work on environmental factors related to schizophrenia. Prior to leaving the institute in 1971, Wynne developed his ideas of the deviant communication patterns within families. After becoming chief of the newly created Center for Studies of Schizophrenia in 1968, the Laing-inspired Mosher studied the outcomes of schizophrenics placed in highly supportive, drug-free residential treatment centers. Additionally, in 1970,

NIMH formed the Center for Minority Group Mental Health Programs to improve knowledge of the psychological effects of racism. Only the year before, in the midst of increasingly visible racism within their profession, Black psychiatrists had come together and founded the Black Psychiatrists of America, immediately putting pressure on both NIMH and the American Psychiatric Association to redress racism within their ranks, as well as to allocate resources to the study of the mental health needs of the Black community.

But even while officials declared racism "the number one public health problem facing America today," NIMH was slow to diversify its ranks, staff members (including Kety) disparaged efforts to address "minority problems," and both internal scientists and external grants favored biological research, looking, for instance, at the outcomes of patients put on psychoactive drugs. Researchers routinely championed drugs, even downplaying or creatively reinterpreting data that didn't support pill treatment. For instance, when some found that individuals put on placebo were less likely to be readmitted to a mental hospital, they suggested that hospital staff had corrupted the experiment. Knowing certain patients had been put on a placebo, researchers proposed, staff had overcompensated with special treatment, setting those patients up for better outcomes. NIMH researchers also discouraged use of the word *tranquilizers*, which had negative connotations even without considering the fact that Black Americans were increasingly bearing the brunt of the pill push, following *DSM-II*'s revised criteria.

As psychotropics expanded to target common conditions like anxiety and depression, so did a new theory to explain their mechanism: They corrected a "chemical imbalance" in the brain. In the case of schizophrenia, it was too much dopamine. So claimed a researcher in 1967 after ascertaining that antipsychotics reduced dopamine. According to medical journalist Robert Whitaker, this became the storytelling formula for pharmaceutical companies and their allies for years to come: "Researchers would identify the mechanism of action for a class of drugs, how the drugs either lowered or raised levels of a brain neurotransmitter, and soon the public would be told that people treated with those medications suffered from the opposite problem." Many drug apologists further refused to consider if the pharmacological changes to brain chemistry were negatively impacting patients. Not even after numerous studies found evidence that drug treatment, while initially seeming to stabilize patients, increased the risk of readmission to a psychiatric hospital. The higher the dose, the greater the risk of relapse.

Antipsychotics had yet to prove safe and effective in the long term, and yet state-run psychiatric hospitals were aggressively emptying beds—at least the ones occupied by white patients. Black Americans were more likely to remain institutionalized, as they were perceived to pose a greater threat to society. By 1975, the population of hospitalized individuals was down from 560,000 in 1953 to 193,000. Many who needed intensive treatment had nowhere to go, as the community centers Kennedy had promised either had not materialized or were providing more basic social services than those they required. In some states, including Michigan, funds meant for community centers were used to build or enhance private facilities.

Civil lawsuits and a major change in social policy accelerated deinstitutionalization. Presenting forced hospitalization as a civil rights violation, progressive activists successfully sued states for confining patients against their will, which frightened state administrators into emptying more beds. Then, as part of his Great Society program, President Lyndon B. Johnson secured passage of the Social Security Act Amendments, which established Medicare and Medicaid (health insurance for the elderly and poor, respectively).

These programs did not pay benefits to people living in public institutions, who were already receiving needed care. Before long, state lawmakers realized that Medicare and Medicaid monies could replace their own expenditure on such elderly and sick people, if only they funneled them to for-profit hospitals or nursing homes, which were now cropping up everywhere to receive government payments. To off-load patients, several states passed laws expressly forbidding public hospitals from admitting patients over the age of sixty-five. Others adopted new policies to exclude the elderly. In California, which was especially aggressive in discharging patients, Governor Ronald Reagan was receiving sizable campaign contributions from nursing home industry executives. Similar conflicts of interest arose in other states where patients were being purged.

When Social Security Disability Insurance (SSDI) became available to younger Americans with mental disturbances in the 1970s, state hospitals had an excuse to wash their hands of this population as well. Hospital administrators figured younger patients could use SSDI income for outpatient, private care. Conditions at the newly established private mental hospitals and nursing homes were largely abysmal, as administrators bypassed licensing requirements and operated free of state supervision. Sociologist Andrew Scull observed in 1981, "The logic of the marketplace suffices to ensure that the operators have every incentive to warehouse their charges as cheaply as possible, since the volume of profit is inversely proportional to the amount expended on the inmates."

An average day for a patient included sleeping, eating, smoking, watching television, and staring out the window. There was no meaningful care plan. For elderly patients, the transfer from public to private institutions often yielded premature death. When the number of transfers exceeded the capacity of private establishments, many found themselves in settings even less equipped to support them: group houses, foster care homes, halfway houses, room-and-board facilities, and welfare hotels. In many cases, they ceased taking their medications, presenting at emergency rooms in such numbers that they began to be described as having "revolving door syndrome." Kennedy's idea that discharged patients would continue treatment of any sort without designated support persons was proving to be incredibly naive, as was Johnson's faith in for-profit health care.

The lucky ones had family to take them in. Edna, Wilma, and Helen Morlok were among the fortunate, always having their mother's home when they relapsed, couldn't hold down a job, or were booted from Northville, which had begun to trim its budget. This must have come as a relief to Rosenthal, who kept an eye on the women who'd advanced his career. Except for time spent abroad, he made a point to visit Lansing twice a year throughout the 1960s and '70s. He'd drive out there with Olive Quinn and stay for two days at a time to see that the sisters, by then in their thirties and forties, were holding it together. In between visits, the quadruplets and their mother wrote letters to give updates. If one of them fibbed or withheld important information, the others always made the truth known. Edna also got in the habit of calling Rosenthal whenever the voices were really distressing her. He always found time to listen and offer ideas for how she might cope.

While Sarah had been living in DC, Rosenthal had even once invited her over to his house for dinner. "I can picture it very clearly," his son, Scott, remembers. "I sat in one corner, she the opposite. She was shy. Very polite. As kids, we got a kick out of the fact that she called him Dr. Rosenthal."

After the publication of the book, Rosenthal's children saw him become somewhat of a celebrity. The newspapers profiled him, and many world-renowned scientists came to the house for dinner.

Among them was Manfred Bleuler, son of Eugen and a psychiatrist in his own right, who'd been "plugging the quads book as though he were collecting royalties," according to a letter Rosenthal had previously sent Dave Shakow. "I could feel the brain power in the room," Rosenthal's youngest daughter, Amy, says, remembering the hours-long conversation over the dinner table at their home in Bethesda. "I was too young to understand anything, but I knew it was important." Long after the last plate was cleared away, she sat to absorb some of the scientists' fervor. "Their enthusiasm was contagious."

Professional societies loaded Rosenthal with honors, and the University of California–Davis offered him a professorship, which he'd seriously considered. But that would have meant forgoing the studies in Jerusalem and then Denmark, which gave his wife and children the experience of a lifetime.

It was on a venture in Europe that the Rosenthal children first saw their father become very angry. The incident made an impression, as they'd never seen him show such emotion. They were trying to ride a ferry back from Germany when Rosenthal got into an argument with the operator, who was wearing a military-style uniform. They were both speaking German, though Rosenthal had a Yiddish grammar. The operator refused to permit them on the ferry, saying it was full. He didn't care that Scott was visibly sick. Even though he was out of sorts, Scott could clearly sense lingering tensions from the war.

It would be another five or six years before Rosenthal's children began to more regularly observe out-of-character behavior on his part—and still another before people outside the family took note. Before that, Rosenthal got his eldest daughter off to college, walked her down the aisle, welcomed a grandson named after him, and led the adult psychology lab through a series of organizational changes, some of which struck his colleagues as questionable, if not terribly concerning.

The institutional reform began in 1972, when two high-ranking research directors at NIMH announced that they expected labs to de-stress psychosocial research in favor of more promising studies in the biological and chemical sciences. "It became a matter of resetting priorities," Parloff explained of the policy handed down by John Eberhart and Robert Cohen. "It was time to recognize that the anticipated contributions of sociology and psychology, especially regarding knowledge about more effective treatment of mental illness, had been disappointing and limited. It now appeared that the important advances were going to be made much more rapidly in the hard rather than the soft sciences." This decision came after NIMH had split from NIH, then temporarily rejoined it, but before it became part of the newly established Alcohol, Drug Abuse, and Mental Health Administration. (In 1992, NIMH was again reabsorbed by NIH, where it remains today.) These realignments reflected budgetary disputes, but also leaders' struggles to delineate the mission of the institute following the so-called Thorazine revolution. Was NIMH going to continue its work in community health or was it going to do basic research?

Perceiving this new directive to mean more targeted and practical research, Rosenthal began to whittle down the scope of his lab to only include subjects he was knowledgeable about. This meant researchers in fields like animal behavior and child development had to move to other departments. Rosenthal also renamed the lab "Psychology and Psychopathology." Some realized these changes were in his own interest. "He didn't want a big lab like Shakow," one colleague recalled. "He didn't want to spend ninety percent of his time being an administrator." Only years later would this colleague and others learn that there was something else going on.

Not even Parloff suspected anything was the matter with his friend until the day Cohen called and asked, "What's going on with Dave?" Cohen proceeded to tell of a strange encounter with Rosenthal. Rosenthal had mentioned that he and Marcia were looking to sell their summer home in western Maryland. When Cohen, who was in the market with his wife to buy, asked him to describe the place, Rosenthal attempted to sketch the layout but couldn't come up with a drawing that remotely resembled the house. He went back to his office to work on the sketch, but he still couldn't come up with anything. On the phone with Parloff, Cohen claimed to be concerned about his conceptual abilities.

"That's ridiculous," said Parloff. "You know, Dave lives right down the street from us, and I see him often. There's nothing wrong with him."

He hung up the phone feeling aggrieved for his friend. Then he thought back to an incident he'd witnessed between Rosenthal and his wife while the two had been over at his house. Rosenthal had behaved badly toward Marcia, though Parloff hadn't thought much of it at the time. As Rosenthal had recently undergone retinal surgery, he figured it was an unfortunate reaction to stress. Could it be more than that?

By the late '70s, other lab chiefs at NIMH were finding Rosenthal too disorganized to collaborate with. They couldn't count on him to meet deadlines or fulfill his part of projects, so they began to rely less and less on the lab. At one point, a colleague named Virgil Carlson reached out to Marcia to see if he could stop by the house and visit. "Oh no," she replied. "If anybody he knows from the lab comes to visit him, he goes into a tantrum after they leave. He just can't stand that. It makes him really upset. It's far better if you don't come and see him."

At that point, Rosenthal had begun to drive so erratically that his children refused to get into the car with him. Laura vividly remembers him trying to drive her and her newborn son while visiting them at their new home in North Carolina. "I was terrified. I wouldn't let him." Like Parloff, they'd seen him get short with their mother, which had never been his way. He'd always respected her, treating her as an intellectual equal. He was also getting lost in his neighborhood. After walking to and from work for two decades, he could no longer remember the route. Sometimes he would figure it out after a few detours. Other times a friend would see him and walk him home, graciously pretending it was just for conversation's sake. According to his son, no one ever said anything, but they "had to know"—the scientist who'd won international acclaim for his study of the mind was now losing his own.

Chapter Thirteen

Edna had put on a good face for Sarah's wedding in 1961, but the truth was she'd been as furious as Cain when he went after his brother Abel in the field. She'd been brought up as the most accomplished daughter, but ever since graduation, Sarah's star had shone the brightest. And if marriage wasn't already a difficult act to follow, her sister had gone and had a baby.

On December 8, 1963, Sarah delivered a boy, William Cotton, at the Royal Air Force Hospital in Mildenhall, England. Four weeks later, the family of three returned to the states for George's next assignment in Grand Forks, North Dakota. Before settling into their new place, Sarah brought her little bundle of joy over to the family home, where Edna was still living. Sadie prepared a big meal and presented Sarah with a baby stroller and clothes. Edna contributed some money to the gifts, even though she felt less than elated for her sister. Sarah stayed with them for two months before joining her husband in North Dakota.

It wasn't long after this that Edna began to pursue a neighbor. Charles ("Chuck") Van Sickle was an older, married man whose children had been schoolmates of the quadruplets. He owned a dance studio and workshop, earning good money from these businesses as well as his salary as a chief engineer for a local plant. Once the two of them became sexual partners, Edna demanded that he favor her over his own family, including his daughter who worked at the studio as a dance instructor. Perhaps in her heart of hearts, it was her desire for this man to replace Carl, in whose eyes she'd always been number one.

When Edna first showed an interest in Chuck, Sadie was highly disturbed. She told David Rosenthal and Olive Quinn that she did not approve of her daughter's behavior, even if she trusted the neighbor to be a gentleman. But after the affair developed, she grew to tolerate it, as Chuck was rather useful to an aging woman like herself. He brought groceries to the house, helped with household maintenance, and chauffeured them to Detroit to visit Wilma and Helen, who were still living in a halfway house and state hospital, respectively. He would also come over and put Edna to bed for her. Over time, she even began to wonder if the arrangement would help Edna to acclimate to men, eventually giving her the confidence to date people more suited for marriage. Though she was now in her thirties, Edna had never gone on a proper date.

According to Sadie, Mrs. Van Sickle was remarkably accepting of the liaison. She once told Sadie that her husband always liked to have some protégé and it was far better for him to spend his time and money on them than some hoodlum. In her mind, the association was "helpful to him." She might have felt differently if there was a chance of Edna becoming pregnant. But at her request, Chuck had been sterilized after the birth of his fourth child.

For all her investment in the affair, Edna did not actually enjoy sex and often felt such guilt over it that she became ill. She periodically took sick leave from her job at a local office of the Internal Revenue Service. When she became too debilitated for this work, she decided to teach dance at the studio. This panned out all right at first, but she soon found Chuck's appetites to be overwhelming.

All this time, Mrs. Van Sickle was counseling her on the ways of life. She seemed to want Edna to succeed almost as much as Sadie, who had a formal plan to help her three ailing daughters return to public life. First Sadie was going to help Edna get on her feet so that she could live independently or at least tolerate others' company. Only at that point would she arrange for Wilma to move from the halfway house into the family home, where this daughter could have Mother's full attention. When Wilma became well and moved out, the chronically hospitalized Helen could be discharged and have her chance. It had taken decades, but Sadie finally seemed to understand that, in failing to view her daughters as individuals, she may have contributed to their troubles, and the only thing to do now was to treat them as only children.

Sometimes, when speaking with Rosenthal and Quinn, Sadie grew sad at the discussion of her past ways of doing things. But she refused to admit that she'd ever favored one daughter over another and always reassured them—or rather herself—that she'd done her best.

Sadie's plans fell apart when Wilma became well enough to come home before Edna could handle another sister. While she dreaded having both in the house at once, there was no other option. Only a few months later, she received a letter from George containing a photograph of Sarah and her baby. One look at her married daughter and she could see that she'd relapsed into her own troubled state. Worried that Sarah was not fit to care for her child, she arranged for her and the baby to come home. During their visit, she learned that her son-in-law was spending most of his off-duty hours at the bar. When George came to Lansing for a few days, she observed him squander money on liquor and gambling while his son was in threadbare clothes.

Edna initially protested Sarah's coming. She accused her sister of trying to drive her out of the house with her son and all his noise. Upon seeing Sarah in trouble, she softened a bit. She even offered to take her nephew for walks when Sarah wasn't up for the task.

When push came to shove, the quadruplets always bore one another's burdens. But the company ultimately proved too much for Edna to handle. In 1967, she was readmitted to NIMH, this time only for treatment. She stayed for three and a half months, during which time Wilma took up with Chuck, who'd tried to warn Edna against seeking psychiatric help. He thought poorly of shrinks.

Sarah and William ended up living at home for several years, as George was deployed to Taipei, Taiwan, where there was no possibility of joining him. It wasn't until he was assigned to Japan to conduct air crash rescue in Vietnam that they were reunited.

Before Sarah departed for what would be a two-year trip, Edna gave her a travel diary. Maybe Edna hoped she would fill these pages with her exploits, instead of writing jealousy-inducing missives about them. While at NIMH, she'd tried to duplicate Sarah's success for herself. Her mother had egged her on, saying if she went back to the institute, she could become well like Sarah had. On Sundays in Bethesda, she'd ridden a bus downtown to Luther Place, where Sarah had fallen in love. She was so invested in catching up with her sister that she regressed if Sadie ever related bad news about Sarah. She once told her psychiatrist at the Clinical Center that Sarah represented the goal she was trying to reach, so if Sarah was cracking up, her own prospects were shaky.

Night after night in Japan, Sarah did write in the diary about the beautiful countryside and the many hobbies she was taking up: geisha-doll making, flower arranging, and lapidary. In August 1969, when William was five and now going by Bill, she had an even greater occasion to recount: the birth of her second son, David.

For the rest of her life, Edna would swear to having sympathetic labor pains half a world away. She'd claim to have been debilitated by abdominal pain, headache, and vomiting in the hours before George's father called to share the good news, at which point she got up and felt fine again. She and her sisters had always believed that twins could feel each other's pain, which may not have surprised anyone, given how symbiotically involved with each other they were. But there was also, undoubtedly, something of an expressed wish in Edna's memories of labor—a wish to become the sister who had eclipsed her.

It's not hard to imagine Edna daydreaming of a baby to call her own, in her moments alone, even drifting upstairs for her old doll and rocking it in her arms as she shushed it back to sleep. Not only was she consumed by her yearnings, she had never been "brought up on reality—all pretense." Such were the words of an old family friend who had spoken with NIMH investigators in the 1950s. "Pretend they are rich, pretend they are invited to high-class parties," the unnamed man said of Carl and Sadie. "And the parents got the girls pretending."

This particular man had seen a rare glimpse of the family when he stopped by their home on Christmas Eve in 1954, just before they left for NIMH. The sorry state of the household—it was essentially a madhouse—got him thinking about how the quadruplets had been exploited by their parents, who appeared to be quite jealous of their daughters. He was only quoted speaking of Carl and Sadie's efforts to maintain their celebrity status, but as the NIMH researchers knew, the family fakery was far more extensive.

As Rosenthal put it, there was always an "immanent opposition" between what one said, did, think, or felt. In fact, there was so much irrationality that he thought the family's case vividly illustrated (not to mean proved) the theory that schizophrenia was learned. How families learned to be irrational was not something *The Genain Quadruplets*, nor the midcentury psychiatric establishment, had really explored—they just *were*. But by the 1970s, a growing number of scholars were yoking familial dysfunction to societal dysfunction, creating a framework that could have helped to paint a fuller picture of the quadruplets' world, if anyone had been motivated to apply it.

Anthropologist Jules Henry, for instance, insisted that schizophrenic children learned to "sham" (pretend) from their parents, who themselves moved in a world defined by shamming. "It is clear that our civilization is a tissue of contradictions and lies," Henry wrote in 1967, marveling that anyone could be sane in the modern day. The United States was particularly adept at inducing both clinical and more generalized psychosis in its people, thanks to its rampant racism and militarism. Henry decried as an "outstanding example of social sham" the "condition of the Negro, who lives like a rat, being told he lives in a democracy and that everything is being done to improve his lot." Black-led riots were merely expressions of hostility in the face of sham. "On the international scene," Henry went on, "the biggest sham is the war in Vietnam, where the United States, while proclaiming to the world that it is building a nation, is destroying one."

Such a theory attempted to bring together Henry's ethnographic observations of families with one clinically psychotic child and his wider observations of American culture. He was clearly influenced by the civil rights activists who were drawing on the language of madness. Besides King, Malcolm X had declared insanity a sane response to racism. There was also the social critic and literary icon James Baldwin, who observed in 1963 that Black children "[ran] the risk of becoming schizophrenic" in public schools, as the idea that the nation defended "liberty and justice for all" totally belied their lived experience. White people, in Baldwin's mind, suffered even more, as they truly believed the "collection of myths." (This was one reason Black Americans could feel so little hatred toward their oppressors—they tended to dismiss them "as the slightly mad victims of their own brainwashing.") That both Baldwin and Malcolm X bypassed the family, making *America* the schizophrenogenic mother, while Henry tried to keep both in view probably had much to do with the disparate political functions of white and Black families in the United States.

Over in England, the Scottish psychoanalyst R. D. Laing elaborated upon Bateson's double bind to draw other links between family and society—in this way, also centering whiteness in the formation of pathology. In his 1967 book, *The Politics of Experience and The Bird of Paradise*, Laing explored the rather violent ways the modern family molded members into obedient citizens by putting them in knots. The function of the family was "to promote respect, conformity, obedience; to con children out of play; to induce a fear of failure; to promote respect for work; to promote respect for 'respectability.'" In most cases, the family successfully manipulated children into supporting these virtues, which corresponded with cruel political and social policies, such as nuclear armament. These families were known as normal. But in other cases, one or more family members told the ugly truth about society using garbled language and other idioms of fools. These individuals were often diagnosed as schizophrenic. To make the case for a more politicized psychoanalysis, Laing revived the work of Austrian analyst Wilhelm Reich, who had identified sexual repression within the family as the primary mechanism of authoritarianism. For Reich, Germans had chosen Nazism over communism precisely because nineteenth-century child-rearing tactics had succeeded in rendering them so obedient and afraid.

American feminists were also analyzing the family as a social institution. It was this group—and particularly, a woman named Florence Rush—who finally forced the public to acknowledge pervasive child sexual abuse. In an April 1971 speech delivered at a conference on rape, Rush challenged the commonly held view that child abusers were psychologically deviant, positing that abusers were actually everyday men who wielded unchecked power over women and children in the off-limits domain of the family. If society was serious about eradicating the harm of children, it needed to reform the nuclear family and compel fathers to share equally in the care of children. For these bold claims, along with her confession to have been abused by an uncle and a dentist in childhood, Rush received a standing ovation. The National Organization of Women then took up her call, throwing its energies into the passage of a congressional bill, sponsored by Minnesota senator Walter Mondale, that would have funded an expansion of children's services, including day care with sliding fees. President Nixon swiftly vetoed the bill, citing its "family-weakening implications." He subsequently signed a child abuse prevention bill that divorced abuse from the social problems that gave rise to it, instead providing grants to states to support the prevention, investigation, and prosecution of cases. This better suited a president who positioned himself as a defender of law and order.

In 1975, a new edition of the popular reference manual *Comprehensive Textbook of Psychiatry* made no mention of the psychological effects of sexual abuse and stated that familial incest occurred at an estimated rate of one in a million. But Rush refused to let the matter go. In 1977, she published an essay in *Chrysalis* that took Sigmund Freud and his profession to task for sweeping abuse under the rug. This piece, titled "The Freudian Coverup," asked why Freud had distanced himself from his original seduction theory and come to view his patients' sexual memories as fantasies. Rush was certain he had been right the first time, only revising his ideas out of cowardice. Because of his actions, Western society had managed to keep repressed the nasty truth at its core.

For all her indignation, Rush took care to accentuate Freud's Victorian-ness and de-judaize him, according to scholar Eli Bromberg. As a Jewish woman herself, she surely understood the ethno-racial stakes of charging him with the cover-up of incest, as did the Jewish feminists whom she inspired. With the exception of Betty Friedan's *The Feminine Mystique*, Jewish-authored books addressing abuse conspicuously excommunicated Freud, which helped their authors and a good many Jewish men—not just the father of psychoanalysis—to disappear into whiteness. Because Black feminists addressing sexual abuse did not engage in the same protective politics, Black men became disproportionately pathologized by second-wave literature. Thus, even an effort to recognize the universality of sexual abuse became bogged down by the usual stereotypes about who embodied innocence and who was a menace.

Rush nevertheless succeeded in forcing the issue of child molestation into the public square, and her work further illuminates what the contributors to *The Genain Quadruplets* could not quite see: Society, and not just the quadruplets' family, was deeply troubled. While these contributors frowned upon Carl and Sadie's "sadistic" decision to circumcise Helen and Wilma, and even the "psychopathic surgeon" who cut into them, they did not dwell on the fact that the procedure had been forced upon countless so-called sex addicts around the country. And while they condemned Carl's sex games, if not exactly grasping their impact, they regarded such games as the doings of a madman, rather than a society that expressed racial anxieties as sexual ones, rendering many minds pornographic.

The quadruplets were formed in a world gone mad. Some, like Laing, might have said this fact disproved their own diagnoses, as if only people *or* worlds could be pathological—as if only medical scientists *or* social theorists could speak with authority about madness. But was it possible that both camps had something to say about the realms of pain and distress that consumed the four women? Could it be that the thing society called mental illness was far too heterogeneous for any single discipline to describe it?

Ever since the days when scientific men had jockeyed against priests for jurisdiction over the mad, there had been partisans loudly proclaiming their grand theories of everything and steamrolling all contrary views. The 1960s and '70s were no exception. Perturbed that psychiatry had succeeded in reframing moral and social struggles ("problems in living") as medical ones, the Hungarian American psychiatrist Thomas Szasz declared mental illness "a myth," also denouncing state-sponsored treatment with alarming stories of the Soviets' uses of psychiatry for the purposes of thought control. (In the libertarian Szasz's view, only private psychotherapy was justified.) But as Freud had keenly understood, just because symptoms had moral or social valences it did not mean they were not pathological. British social theorist Peter Sedgwick made this same point when he wrote in response to Szasz that mental illness "is to be sure, a social status: but before that, it is a private hell." For critics like Sedgwick, so-called anti-psychiatrists' attacks on government-funded psychiatric treatment were especially problematic, as they presented all public psychiatry as an exercise of state power when, in reality, governments were directing psychiatrists to discharge even those patients who desired treatment.

Indeed, in Ronald Reagan's America, the true plight of the mentally ill was not being mind-controlled but left for dead in the streets. Soon after assuming the Oval Office in 1981, the Gipper slashed federal benefits for many disabled Americans amid racially coded allegations of welfare fraud. On the campaign trail, Reagan had popularized the character of the "welfare queen," the lazy, inner-city (Black) woman who lived off the largesse of honest, hardworking (white) taxpayers. In office, he continued to blow this and other racist dog whistles as part of a broader GOP strategy to win over southern Democrats. As later outlined by his adviser Lee Atwater, conservative politicians calculated that they only had to drop the word *nigger* for more respectable slogans like *cutting taxes* and *states' rights*—everyone inferred these policies would disproportionately harm Black Americans, who were trying to gain their footing after nearly four hundred years of slavery and Jim Crow. Whites within and beyond the South rallied around the new president's plan to shrink the federal government, likely unaware that they or their loved ones would pay a steep price for the retrenchment of social programs.

Following the cancellation of their benefits, hundreds of thousands of mentally ill and other disabled Americans were without income to spend on housing or private treatment. Making matters worse, the "public option" was being gutted. The Omnibus Budget Reconciliation Act of 1981 repealed most of the Mental Health Systems Act of 1980, which President Jimmy Carter had signed only a few months previously in order to provide funding for existing community mental health centers. The dollars were diverted to the military and soon-to-be-privatized jails and prisons.

In the wake of the funding cuts, the American Psychiatric Association expressed particular concern for schizophrenics, and others lamented that those with serious mental illness were joining the ranks of the homeless. One of these was sixty-one-year-old Rebecca Smith, a former college valedictorian who captured headlines after freezing to death in a makeshift cardboard shelter in New York City. As news coverage of tragedies like Smith's spiked, the Reagan administration blamed a culture of dependency for any seeming rise in homelessness. "I think some people are going to soup kitchens voluntarily," said White House adviser Edwin Meese. "I know we've had considerable information that people go to soup kitchens because the food is free and that's easier than paying for it." The president echoed this sentiment, saying people slept on grates "by choice."

By starving health and welfare programs while simultaneously feeding for-profit prisons, the Reagan administration resurrected a society wherein people with serious mental illness were put behind bars for lack of any other institution to "care" for them. Reaganism further transformed the lives of the mentally ill by crushing research on the social determinants of distress. Seeming to recognize how the soft sciences threatened his gospel of personal responsibility (by exposing how human beings were inextricably bound up with one another), Reagan only spared the budgets for natural scientists, which in the psychiatric field included those looking for pathology in the brain. By the 1980s, those on the hunt for a mental illness gene or cluster of genes were still empty-handed, but new brain imaging technologies had shed light on different types of brain damage and biochemical abnormalities, which many believed to be genetically determined. The technologies quickly yielded many new hypotheses for schizophrenia's manifestation. These so excited NIMH researchers that in summer 1981, a few months following Rosenthal's retirement, they brought the Morlok family back to the Clinical Center as outpatients.

Over the course of two weeks, researchers led by Dr. Allan

Mirsky, who had just been appointed lab chief, administered a battery of cognitive and neurobiological tests on the sisters, now fifty-one years old. Sadie, George, and Sarah's two sons, aged eleven and seventeen, also came along, participating in a few tests themselves. Then the quadruplets went to St. Elizabeths Hospital for a six-week, drug-free evaluation that included regular blood, urine, lumbar puncture, and adrenal testing. Sarah also had to be weaned off medication as she'd gone on an antipsychotic in 1976, following a psychotic episode and suicide attempt. She'd tried to overdose on prescription medications.

The tests were cumbersome, especially the spinal tap. None of the sisters were pleased to have a needle jabbed into their backs. David Cotton, Sarah's younger son, vividly remembers being tested himself. As a kid, he'd resented having dozens of wires attached to his skull so the people in white coats could find some deep dark secret about him. "They acted like I was some prodigy for future studies," he reminisces. The investigators also took samples of his blood.

In David's recollection, none of the NIMH researchers really probed into his life during the 1981 stay, even though they knew it was uneasy. His mother had told them that social services had removed both him and his brother from the home after visiting and finding neglect. She'd been dealing with her own crises, and their father was nowhere to be found. Then there'd been the incident at the hotel in Bethesda, which Mirsky had resolved. For whatever reason—David doesn't remember—he and his older brother had been given their own room. Being unsupervised, the two boys had gotten into all kinds of mischief. First, they'd gone around the hotel and stolen soda pop from all the vending machines. Then they'd chucked objects from their room into an open pool in the atrium. Ashtrays, lamps, whatever they could get their hands on. The hotel workers had been livid, but then Mirsky had come and smoothed things over.

Rosenthal's successor and his crew were testing a number of hypotheses: the "dopamine hypothesis" (schizophrenia was connected to excess dopamine in the brain); the "norepinephrine hypothesis" (schizophrenia, particularly the paranoid type, was connected to excessive norepinephrine in the brain); the "enzymatic defect hypothesis" (schizophrenia corresponded to low enzymes for the metabolism of major neurotransmitters); the "endogenous hallucinogen hypothesis" (the production of phenylethylamine or dimethyltryptamine produced symptoms); the "viral hypothesis" (a viral infection of the central nervous system was implicated in the development of schizophrenia); and the "autoimmune hypothesis" (antibodies directed against the brain produced schizophrenia). If proved, any of these hypotheses would obviate concerns about life stressors—or so many were beginning to think. If, for instance, schizophrenia presented as excess dopamine in parts of the brain and dopamine levels could be altered with drug treatment, did it really matter what circumstances had brought on the condition? Such logic hailed back to Freud, who'd implied that the psychic action between analyst and analysand was all that mattered. But it was surely also a sign of the times that scientists truly believed they could situate battered people outside of time, place, and politics.

Lynn E. DeLisi, Allan F. Mirsky, Monte S. Buchsbaum, et al. published the first of a three-paper series on the quadruplets in *Psychiatry Research* in 1984. Off medication, the women did not appear to have excess dopamine, nor did they have unusual concentrations of norepinephrine. They also did not have significantly lower activity of monoamine oxidase, thought to support the dopamine and norepinephrine hypotheses. There were no positive antibody titers in the cerebrospinal fluid for viruses believed to be associated with schizophrenia, and only one of the quadruplets had a positive antinuclear antibody titer, making the autoimmune hypothesis "unlikely to be relevant to any inherited component of their illness."

Dopamine beta-hydroxylase (DBH), the enzyme that converts dopamine to norepinephrine and phenylethylamine to phenylethanolamine, *was* lower in all quadruplets, as well as their non-schizophrenic family members. (The researchers noted that while one population study found low DBH to be common among schizophrenics, other studies, including by DeLisi, found otherwise; they also noted that the decrease could be related to chronic medication use, as indicated by previous studies.) The sisters' platelet alpha-adrenergic receptor numbers were notably increased, and PGE1-stimulated cAMP production was reduced. According to researchers, both alterations were previously observed in chronic schizophrenics. Two of the three biological family members also had increased alpha receptor concentrations, and one had decreased PGE1-stimulated cAMP production. Potentially due to another genetic alteration and illness marker, the quadruplets and their mother had high levels of urinary phenylethylamine excretion. DeLisi and her colleagues admitted they could not specifically define the genetic aspects of schizophrenia in the quadruplets' case, but were nevertheless stirred by their discoveries, which they hoped would yield others.

In the second paper for *Psychiatry Research*, Buchsbaum and his colleagues reported on neurological findings. The sisters' computed tomography (CT) scans were normal, showing no evidence of ventricular enlargement and little atrophy. In a brainstem auditory evoked responses (BAERs) diagnostic, the sisters did show slowed conduction time, indicating possible brainstem dysfunction. But there was no meaningful differentiation among them, even though the severity of their conditions varied. This meant that the differences in their outcomes could not be attributed to the amount of brain damage, at least as detected by then-available imaging methods.

Mirsky et al. published a third article comparing the sisters' performance on attention and related tests in both the 1950s and 1980s. This paper attributed their overall improvement on these tests to medication.

Four years later, in 1988, Mirsky and Olive Quinn synthesized the three studies for *Schizophrenia Bulletin*, moving even further away from Rosenthal's hypothesis. Here they wrote that, while differential life experiences could have impacted the severity of the quadruplets' disorders, "biological factors could also have contributed to the variable outcome among the Genains." By this, they primarily meant brain injuries at birth that had yet to be detected. Being the firstborn, Edna would likely have sustained the most traumatic injury, clearing the way for the others. And being the runt, Helen was probably also disproportionately traumatized by passage through the birth canal. This would explain why these two sisters declined considerably (as measured by neuropsychiatric evaluations) when taken off medication, while Sarah actually improved and Wilma appeared to remain intact.

Reflecting on researchers' hyper-focus on the brain, David is bewildered. In his mind, there was so much more to him and his family members that investigators did not bother to capture. If they'd tried to understand his life, he might have told them there'd been times he, too, didn't want to live. Before going to NIMH, he'd tried to kill himself, breaking into a medicine cabinet at a home for troubled youth. And if they had really pried, he might even have offered that he'd been molested. Carl Morlok was dead and gone, but the little clapboard two-story on East Saginaw Street was still a haunting place. The sins of the father had become those of the daughters—some of them, anyway—and then it had been *his* little body that quivered at others' touch. Far from providing asylum, foster care had brought new terrors.

But the NIMH investigators were busy barking up another tree and he was deeply ashamed of his secrets, so he kept them to himself.

Chapter Fourteen

At first, David Rosenthal refused to admit anything was seriously the matter. He'd walk around the house with a book, even though he couldn't make sense of the words. He would fumble with his tie in front of the mirror until his wife came and knotted it for him. He would go to his office at NIMH and shuffle papers around his desk. Frustrated that he wasn't getting any work done but unwilling to think of retiring, he began to go in late and come home early. "He was probably horrified," Scott Rosenthal says of his father's denial of his Alzheimer's disease. "He didn't want to believe it, even though he diagnosed himself."

In 1977, Rosenthal went and saw a specialist in New York who confirmed he had the degenerative brain disease. Only Amy was still at home, as Scott was now a senior in college and Laura was already living in North Carolina. "At that point, my sisters and I knew something was wrong. It hadn't been addressed out loud within the family, but we knew."

Rosenthal soon became too obviously impaired to hold his position as lab chief. In 1980, years after other NIMH scientists had begun to rely on other labs for projects, he was asked to step down, but given an office in the building for his research. This may have been pure charity for the man who had given twenty-five years to the institute, in addition to bringing it worldwide acclaim. After all, no one could have expected him to meaningfully contribute to the work of the lab. Then again, it may have been Rosenthal's enduring charisma that made his colleagues want to keep him around. According to both his daughters, his warmth and kindness outlasted his ability to follow certain conversations, and knowing this, he'd learned to rely on his social graces to buy himself some time. In any case, Rosenthal only managed to go into the office for one year following his demotion before even this became too difficult. Ordinary conversation was impossible, as he often couldn't recall basic facts; and the mechanisms he'd developed to mask his limitations were eroding. In 1981, he officially retired from NIMH.

Letters poured in from adoring colleagues. People were too polite to mention the circumstances for his departure, instead praising his collegiality and contributions to the field. Privately, many were in disbelief about the beloved man's misfortune. "I always thought that only Dave Rosenthal would make it and would dedicate [his books to] people who died too soon," Robert Cohen later told NIMH documentarians. "It was a heartbreaking experience... he was such a remarkable man." Cohen and others made a point to occasionally call the house to check in with Rosenthal. They wanted him to know he wasn't forgotten.

But in his absence, Rosenthal *was* beginning to be forgotten. According to Cohen, his "name got lost with his illness. So many people began to talk about [the quadruplets] as Seymour Kety's study." And following Allan Mirsky's appointment as lab chief, many were eager to move on from Rosenthal's period of tenure. If the lab was going to survive, it needed to be reconstituted, either by reintegrating the sections that Rosenthal had cut or repairing relationships with external researchers. Mirsky seemed up for this task and also that of modernizing the lab to emphasize the brain sciences.

While Mirsky worked to bring the laboratory into the future, Rosenthal continued to deteriorate. When Marcia could no longer keep him busy around the house, even with Amy's help, she enrolled him in adult day care. Every morning a bus would come by the house and take him to the Hebrew Center in Rockville, Maryland, where he would partake in occupational and other forms of therapy. "He was just disappearing right before our eyes," says Scott. Soon he couldn't even dress or feed himself, and few outside the family seemed to understand what was going on, as Alzheimer's disease was not familiar beyond medical-scientific circles. "Oh, he's senile?" people would ask, hearing of his diagnosis. "Forgetting things?"

In 1982, shortly after Amy had left town, Marcia had little choice but to put her husband in residential care. She chose for him to live in Perry Point, the veterans' hospital where the two had met each other all those years ago. The facility was "as good as you could hope for," according to Scott, who lived locally. It was clean and well staffed, but the condition of patients still made it an awfully sad place to be. "There were people wandering around without a clue."

While Rosenthal was at Perry Point, the Danish-American adoption studies came under new scrutiny. Evolutionary geneticist Richard Lewontin, neurobiologist Steven Rose, and psychologist Leon Kamin closely examined the data that Kety had used for a 1975 follow-up study, which again looked for disorder in the biological families of schizophrenic adoptees, but in a much broader population and using interviews, not hospital records, to diagnose relatives. They found that the Danish-American researchers had made a grave mistake in assuming both in 1968 and 1975 that schizophrenic (index) adoptees and control adoptees were placed in equal environments. They came to this stance after finding that in 83 percent of cases where a "soft spectrum" biological relative of an index adoptee had been identified—that is, someone with latent or borderline schizophrenia—there were also "outside the spectrum" diagnoses, such as alcoholism, psychopathy, and syphilitic psychosis. The fact that adoptees' biological families had socially stigmatized conditions struck them as noteworthy because of the universal phenomenon of placement bias.

As Lewontin, Rose, and Kamin explained in their 1984 book *Not in Our Genes*, "The children placed into homes by adoption agencies are never placed randomly." The biological children of college-educated mothers tend to be placed with adoptive parents of higher socioeconomic and educational status, while the children of grade school dropouts tend to be placed into much lower-status adoptive homes. For this reason, it seemed reasonable to ask: "Into what kinds of adoptive homes are infants born into families shattered by alcoholism, criminality, and syphilitic psychosis likely to be placed? Further, might not the adoptive environment into which such children are placed cause them to develop schizophrenia?"

When the three authors examined the adoptive families of schizophrenic and control adoptees, they found that 24 percent of schizophrenic adoptees had an adoptive parent who had been in a mental hospital. None of the adoptive parents of control adoptees had a record of hospitalization. This suggested a possible environmental interpretation of Kety and his colleagues' findings, as the "fact that one's adoptive parent goes into a mental hospital clearly does not bode well for the psychological health of the environment in which one is reared."

Combing through data Kety had provided them, Lewontin, Rose, and Kamin stumbled across another concerning finding: Several of the interviews of index and control adoptees' relatives used for the 1975 study seemed never to have taken place. Instead, they appeared to have been fabricated by the Danish researchers before being analyzed by American diagnosticians for the follow-up paper, in which Kety put "inadequate personality" outside the spectrum, otherwise preserving the broad definition of schizophrenia. When Lewontin, Rose, and Kamin corresponded with one of the Danish researchers about this, the researcher admitted to answering interview questions on behalf of some of the relatives who had died or were unavailable. In one case, a pseudo-interview had been prepared for a biological mother who had died by suicide long before anyone tried to locate her. She had actually been hospitalized twice and diagnosed each time as manic-depressive. Her hospital records had been edited so as to conceal this fact from those analyzing them in 1968. Even by Kety's standards, manic depression (now bipolar disorder) was very clearly outside the schizophrenic spectrum. Thus, Lewontin, Rose, and Kamin could "only marvel" how American diagnosticians managed to decide—not once, but twice—"that she really belonged within the shifting boundaries of the spectrum."

Even without their correspondence with a Danish researcher, the made-up interviews would have come to light. The same year that *Not in Our Genes* was published, American psychologists Kenneth S. Kendler and Alan M. Gruenberg released their own analysis of Kety et al.'s 1975 study, in which they noted funny business. Kendler and Gruenberg, who'd undertaken the analysis to apply the diagnostic criteria of the subsequently published *DSM-III*, wrote that it was easy to discern between "a real interview with a control adoptee" and a "pseudo interview with an index adoptee."

The revelation of the phony interviews and other of the studies' flaws would raise questions about the integrity of the researchers' conclusions in the minds of some experts, though not Kendler and Gruenberg, who actually found the studies sound enough. Seven years later, psychiatrist Peter Breggin would suggest that the genetics of schizophrenia rested on a "house of cards." But a declining Rosenthal would never have the chance to respond to such criticism.

In the late '80s, Marcia was forced to transfer her husband to a private hospital. Reagan-era austerity had led to policy changes at veterans' hospitals, and he was deemed ineligible for care, his illness not being related to military service. She was fortunate to find a private facility of comparable quality—Calvert Manor in Rising Sun, Maryland—but was now saddled with costly bills. According to Scott, she never forgave Reagan for the policies that uprooted her husband from an institute that had meant something to her. Not even when she began to notice a subtle change in his speech and gait, pointing at her television and declaring, "That man has Alzheimer's."

Rosenthal soon became bedridden. He would just lie with a blank stare in his eyes. As much as it pained them, his family continued to visit. Marcia had a theory that if they stopped coming, it would be easier for staff to neglect him. In February 1996, while she was on holiday with her sister in San Antonio, he died. By the time she made it back to the East Coast, the body had been taken for burial. She never cried, claiming to have "no more tears."

Crowds swarmed Rosenthal's funeral ceremony then returned to Scott's house for a reception. Mirsky was there. He was cordial; nevertheless, it was difficult for some of Rosenthal's family members to face the man who had succeeded their loved one. They didn't even know then that Mirsky had taken over the quadruplet studies.

One month after Rosenthal's death and nearly forty years after the investigators had concluded the first study, Mirsky arranged for the Morlok sisters to be studied by NIMH a third time. Years of neoliberal policy had changed the place. The Center for Minority Group Mental Health Programs was now gone, along with the Laingian Loren Mosher. (NIMH dismissed Mosher after he became more outspoken about the pharmacological takeover of psychiatry.) In the wake of the Oklahoma City bombing, an executive order mandated changes to the physical campus, which would further diminish the communitarian atmosphere, even if they took some years to complete. If once the campus had been open for anyone to stroll the gardens and let their children play, it would soon resemble a "terrible fortress." Those were Amy's words, referring to the iron gate, armed security guards, and "sad" feel of the place.

NIMH had thoroughly shapeshifted to the times, though it was hardly the only institution to do so. During the 1980s, many Freudian psychiatrists and therapists had been reeling both from the loss of the Freudian paradigm and the breakneck speed of their field's re-biologization; so when the opportunity came along, these professionals, too, had made something of a Faustian bargain. It had the effect of obscuring the trauma endured by the Morlok sisters and millions of others. It wasn't a bargain with the drug industry, but with an arguably even more powerful force in America: the ascendant Religious Right.

Chapter Fifteen

Sometimes when the light was still weak, David Cotton would get out of bed and go fishing with his brother and father. The three of them didn't talk much, just holding their rods and waiting for something to tug. That was all right with David. Being on the water and in his father's good graces made the times special. Most days his father was drunk or on the road.

"He would also beat us," David now remembers. Typically it was because he and Bill had done something mischievous like prank one of their relatives or neighbors. They once ran toilet paper around a public bathroom.

When Bill got older, he began to steal things. Sometimes David would lie and take the blame so his father would whip him instead. Though he was younger by more than five years, he considered himself Bill's protector. "He was not all there. His personality was not normal, and he wouldn't talk unless spoken to." In David's view, Bill had always been eccentric. And then he'd been in a serious accident as a child, which may have caused brain damage. The family had been living near a base in Alexandria, Louisiana, at the time. Bill had crossed the street on his bicycle to check their mailbox when a car struck him. Upon hearing a scream, Sarah came running out the front door. David still remembers the sight of the mangled bicycle, the blood pouring down the road, and the police officers who arrived on the scene and questioned the young couple in the car. The two strangers never did take responsibility for what happened, and a witness refused to testify about what she'd seen. For these reasons, attorneys settled out of court for a mere $1,700 (about $9,000 today). Bill had to do intensive therapy before he could return to school.

Often when David and Bill were up to no good, their mother was at home fretting about the rent or her absent husband. Even with bills piling up, George Cotton spent much of his income at the VFW or other drinking holes. David didn't know it then, but he was also giving away Sarah's possessions. He tried to impress other women by giving them her nice clothes and, in one case, her cherished IBM typewriter. Her mother had helped her to buy it.

When the boys' misdeeds garnered her attention, she wasn't sure how to respond. There was the time David and Bill got a garden hose and filled the car up with water, hoping to make some kind of swimming pool. They were still living in Louisiana then. "She flipped out. She spanked us every fifteen minutes for days. She didn't know when to stop."

Things got a little better when the family returned to Michigan, briefly living at the Morlok family homestead while they looked for their own place. Grandmother Sadie was kind, showing love as she did for David's three aunts, who were "clearly suffering" even more than his mother. This took some of the pressure off Sarah. But there at that house, David endured new terrors. To start, the home had been burgled on two separate occasions. In each, someone had broken in through the side door, where there was a landing and then steps to the kitchen. No one had been harmed, and nothing of value was taken, but the mere knowledge of the invasions was enough to spook him. "I was always scared to go down those steps."

Then there were the bad actors *within* the home. "Wilma and Helen touched me. They'd put their hands down my pants. They'd also take mine and put it down theirs." They only ever did this when no one else was around.

Like many abused children, David was too embarrassed to tell his mother what happened. And like many children of trauma survivors, he knew to tiptoe around her, never daring to tell her anything that might open an old wound or increase her worries. There was another reason he kept quiet: He wanted to let her have her enchanted view of her sisters. "She was very into herself and her family. Their fame—it made her happy." He would keep his dark secret, even if it made him twitch and wet the bed.

David's molestation occurred right around the time that Florence Rush and other feminists were urging the public to acknowledge child sexual abuse, along with sexual harassment and assault in the workplace. Only a few years later, conservatives would respond with their own views of sexual abuse and what it demanded of society: a return to "traditional" family values. As David's case resembled neither the feminist prototype (involving male abuse of a female victim), nor the conservative one in-the-making, social workers and therapists probably wouldn't have known what to do even if he *had* come forward with it sometime after the fact. It would be many years before he came to understand it himself.

David doesn't know if Wilma and Helen ever molested Bill. When he was about nine, and they were living nearby, both boys were taken from the home. Investigators had been alerted that the teenage Bill was delinquent in school. When they came to inspect his living environment, they were aghast to find neither he nor David knew how to use a knife or fork, nor to look after their hygiene. "We were the living version of *The Jungle Book*," says David. "An animal could have raised us better." His grandmother had tried to help as best she could, but she was caring for his aunts while suffering from her own ailments. Nearly in her eighties, Sadie had arthritis and other pain.

Once in state custody, David was introduced to children with antisocial habits, such as smoking, and he eventually took these on. "I would have fared better at home." Sometimes social workers did try to place him back with his mother, but they inevitably decided he didn't have adequate supervision and took him back into the system.

Going to Bethesda in 1981 was something of a reprieve. He loathed being treated like a lab rat, but he'd gotten to be with his brother, who was about to age out of foster care and look for work. His parents were then on the brink of divorce. His mother had hoped family therapy at NIMH would help them to patch things up and even get them to a point where he and Bill could be brought home. Unfortunately, his father hadn't liked the idea of talking to a stranger about their private lives. They went their separate ways, though not officially dissolving the marriage until 1988, at which point George moved to Florida, finding a wife fifteen years his senior. "She had money," David explains. "I think that was what attracted him."

After NIMH, David was in and out of various foster homes, where he was exploited and brutalized in still new ways. "It's human farming," he says of the foster care system. "People make money from it. Even if they go in with the right intentions, they get addicted to money. Once you're eighteen, you're out. That's when the money stops coming." He was always made to feel inferior to any biological children his foster parents had. And he was beaten, even for things beyond his control. He partly attributes the persistence of abuse to the "religious hypocrisy" of the families who took him in. At thirteen, for instance, he still wet the bed; for this, one set of parents made a practice of rubbing his face in the sheets. They acted as though he was morally rotten. But whenever authorities came by the house, they would turn on the charm. "They knew how to keep everything within the home. They would just transform into totally different people. They were all very good at that."

It's possible, when it came to inflicting and then concealing physical abuse, some of these families were influenced by a burgeoning industry of books and media on "biblical" parenting and the rights and duties of parents to punish by force. The 1970s and '80s saw the rise of mega-influencers like evangelical Christian psychologist James Dobson, who founded Focus on the Family and authored a slew of manuals pushing child discipline as the means to combat what he perceived to be the cultural disorder begun in the 1960s with the antiwar and feminist movements.

Dobson's *Dare to Discipline* was particularly influential, quickly selling over two million copies. Published in 1970 while he was still working at the American Institute of Family Relations, a secular eugenics organization founded to promote marriage and reproduction among able-bodied white couples, the book urged that pain was "a marvelous purifier." It wasn't necessary or prudent to be too harsh or incessant with corporal punishment, as "a little bit of pain [went] a long way." Readers could use paddles and switches with "sufficient magnitude to cause the child to cause genuine tears." Those who learned to obey their parents could be expected to obey teachers, police officers, religious men, and other moral authorities, or so he claimed. Dobson followed up this book with *The Strong-Willed Child* in 1978. Here he described beating the recalcitrant family pet dachshund (named after his intellectual hero Sigmund Freud) and then made the point that discipline was even more important with human beings. He also recommended squeezing the trapezius muscle at the back of the neck to control wayward kids and leaving paddles on the dresser to frighten them into obedience.

Similar to the way Freud viewed children as having innate "drives" toward violence against opposite-sex parents, Dobson viewed children as being driven to rebel because of original sin. But whereas Freud advocated talk therapy and greater understanding of the unconscious, Dobson preferred the rod. Children were not young people to be taught, but beasts to be tamed—a notion reminiscent of Victorian-era physician Moritz Schreber, whose translated work Dobson may also have read. Fortunately for Dobson, the Bible was full of passages praising the virtues of corporal punishment. By quoting these passages—and by taking great care to distinguish himself from those *other* (secular) psychologists—he managed to gain the trust of the churchgoing masses.

According to journalist Talia Lavin, who authored a Substack series on Dobson, many millennials who were neck-pinched as kids now report flinching at any touch on the shoulder. Some also describe a series of abusive relationships following their "trauma bonding" in childhood. (The psychologist famously advised readers that they should always explain they only hurt their kids out of love, in that way providing parents a means to cement the emotional bond and prolong the hurt, which often went far beyond a "little bit of pain.")

But Dobson was hardly the only one to persuade parents that God willed for children to be totally submissive. There were also figures like Bill Gothard and Michael Farris, founders of the Institute in Basic Youth Conflicts (formerly Campus Teams and later the Institute in Basic Life Principles) and the Home School Legal Defense Association, respectively. Gothard and his colleagues toured the country delivering seminars on "character education," core parts of which were corporal punishment and rigid submission to patriarchal rule within the Christian home, to audiences of more than twenty thousand. Building on the "dominionist" philosophy of avowed white supremacist R. J. Rushdoony, Gothard did not desire for Christians to permanently retreat from society, but only for them to amass an army that could one day replace liberal democracy with a form of government based on biblical law as they defined it.

Farris, for his part, advised homeschooling and foster parents on ways to fend off pesky social workers who called or stopped by the house, also lobbying lawmakers to deregulate homeschooling and grant foster parents the right to physically punish foster children. He, too, characterized the state as an adversary of parents trying to save their children from decadent society, later going so far as to write a novel dramatizing two families who faced persecution at the hands of the child welfare system and the godless United Nations. Following Reagan's election, paranoia of the-state-as-Antichrist was more intense than ever, even though the Reverend Jerry Falwell and other prominent conservatives were successfully taking control of the halls of government.

It so happened that just as Dobson, Gothard, and Farris were laying the legal and theological groundwork for parents to have unfettered control over their children's bodies, and just as David was being victimized by his aunts and foster parents, the public was entering into another moral panic regarding child sexual abuse. This one, like that of the '30s and '40s, was largely fueled by social anxieties, doing little to protect those who were being harmed or who were vulnerable. By some accounts, it made the abuse crisis worse, as it shrouded cases like David's, where the nature of the abuse didn't serve the broader narrative of civilizational decline. It did so, in part, by binding together the mental health professions and conservative religion more tightly than ever before.

The hullabaloo began in 1980 with the publication of *Michelle Remembers*, an autobiography by Canadian Michelle Smith (real surname Proby) and her psychiatrist-turned-husband Lawrence Pazder, which told of Smith's supposed childhood satanic ritual abuse. The story went like this: An adult Smith was being seen by Pazder for depression following a miscarriage when she confided that she had some horrible dream to relate but could not bring herself to tell it. In a subsequent session, she screamed for twenty-five minutes, convulsed, and assumed the voice of a five-year-old. Over the next fourteen months, Pazder used hypnosis to put her into a childlike state, in which she "recovered" memories of satanic ritual abuse occurring in the 1950s at the hands of Satanists, who'd gained influence over her mother in their hometown of Victoria, British Columbia. Smith's abuse included being locked in a wire cage, subjected to ritual sex abuse, forced to witness an infant sacrifice, and rubbed with human body parts. In the last ritual, lasting eighty-one days in a local cemetery, Jesus and Mary intervened, healing her scars and blocking her memories until the time was right to tell the world what she'd endured.

Shortly after the book's publication, Smith's father claimed she'd manufactured the story out of whole cloth. Reporters could not corroborate the alleged events. There was, for instance, no record of a car crash that Smith claimed to be involved in, nor of a hospital visit for any injuries. A school yearbook showed she'd been photographed on the day she was supposed to be locked in a basement. Nevertheless, *Michelle Remembers* flew off shelves as swiftly as white southerners flocking to lynching trees after one of their own uttered the word *rape*. Catapulted to international fame,

Smith and Pazder traveled the world giving lectures on satanic ritual abuse and recovered memory therapy to law enforcement officials, mental health providers, and clergy. Recently converted to Catholicism, Smith also consulted on many of the satanic ritual abuse cases that came in the book's wake, notably the McMartin preschool trial. That trial is even better remembered for fueling what is now known as the Satanic Panic.

In Manhattan Beach, California, a mother claimed to have found blood in her son's diaper, accusing an employee at his preschool, McMartin, of sodomizing him. Police arrested the man, Raymond Buckey, then let him go for lack of evidence. They then issued a letter to approximately two hundred families asking for any leads. It was a template of "what not to do," according to one contemporary expert. Rather than ask open questions, it planted ideas in parents' heads. Unsurprisingly, parents then interrogated their children, not resting until they heard of wrongdoing. The police hired therapists to interview the children. None of the contracted professionals were trained for this kind of situation, asking many leading questions. Before long, children began to tell of such sensations as a goat man, flying teacher, orgies, child sacrifice, disinterment, and dismemberment, leading police to rearrest Buckey and turn their attention to other employees, including his mother, who owned the school that Buckey's grandmother had founded. Social worker Kee MacFarlane, a former lobbyist of the National Organization for Women, used anatomically correct dolls to interrogate the kids, praising those who reported misdeeds as "smart." She then went before Congress claiming the children were being forced to engage in bizarre rituals involving feces and animals. Shortly afterward, Congress increased funding for child protection programs, much of the money going to conferences and educational literature in which law enforcement officials shared ideas for underhandedly securing guilty convictions, such as by discrediting the defense's witnesses and interviewing children off camera.

Congress also passed the Child Protection Act of 1984, which removed First Amendment protections for child pornography, raised the age of minority from sixteen to eighteen, expanded law enforcement's powers, increased criminal penalties for offenses, and required the attorney general to report to Congress on the prosecutions and convictions of cases. As when Rush had first forced attention to widespread abuse, legislators weren't so interested in the ways patriarchal society encouraged rape or other abuse. According to Richard Beck, who wrote a 2015 book on the McMartin case, *We Believe the Children: A Moral Panic in the 1980s,* they only took to the idea that the country's children were in grave peril, as this perfectly served the narrative that gays and feminists were running amok with their demands for civil liberties. Consequently, while the act put some needed measures in place, it primarily emboldened citizens and law enforcement officers to go after perceived public menaces. In this way, it supplemented such efforts as evangelical beauty queen Anita Bryant's "Save Our Children" campaign, which brandished kids' innocence to promote discrimination against homosexuals in housing, employment, and public services.

Across the nation more than a hundred other white, suburban preschools became the focus of criminal investigation, and individuals collectively lodged more than twelve thousand accusations of organized cult abuse. People alleged that, besides childcare centers, Satanists were using heavy metal music, television, public school teachers, and role-playing games like Dungeons & Dragons to recruit youth.

A network of Christian psychotherapists, psychiatrists, social workers, and exorcists cropped up to support alleged victims, many trying out Smith and Pazder's recovered memory techniques. These religiously inclined professionals helped to infuse therapy with Christian sensibilities while also compelling the secular American Psychiatric Association to recognize multiple personality disorder (MPD) pursuant to ritual abuse in a revised edition of the *DSM-III*, published in 1984. This disorder, now known as dissociative identity disorder (DID), appealed to Christian professionals, because it aligned with their understanding of demonic possession and also allowed them to view their work in terms of a religious crusade. In helping patients to "integrate" personalities, professionals were essentially helping patients to move through sin toward redemption.

Secular professional societies were not oblivious to what was going on. In fact, members of the *DSM-III-R* Advisory Committee on Dissociative Disorders acknowledged that the newly recognized forms of MPD were little more than the "secularized descendants of the Judeo-Christian possession syndrome." In clinical psychologist Richard Noll's summary, these authorities "knew they were expanding the jurisdictional boundary of 'scientific' psychiatry and colonizing the supernatural." But the idea of becoming priest-like was tantalizing, and so psychiatrists claimed for themselves the magical powers once reserved for exorcists. One member of the advisory committee even founded a peer-reviewed journal, *Dissociation*, for scientific investigators to learn about the "hidden holocaust" that was being exacted against the nation's children.

After MPD debuted in the *DSM*, cases of it exploded, with mostly male therapists putting mostly female abuse victims into a childlike state of mind to confess their way to healing. It was the antithesis of the therapeutic approach used for the quadruplets, first at Mercywood and then at NIMH. If, at those institutions, psychiatrists had either minimized the fact that they'd been assaulted or allowed

Edna, Wilma, and Helen to turn away from the clinical gaze, many of these professionals were ready to put rape stories in women's mouths. This was surely reminiscent of Freud's chauvinism, even if the new guard could distinguish themselves from psychoanalysis's founder by claiming to take sexual abuse seriously.

While mental health professionals were morphing into public heroes, traditionalists were using the alleged ritual abuse crisis to discourage mothers from using day care. Moms who *truly* loved their children didn't send them to be sodomized by Satanists, they essentially argued, as if the vast majority of children's abusers did not dwell at home. Despite the overtly anti-feminist rhetoric of the Satanic Panic, many women's rights advocates besides MacFarlane contributed to the hysteria, writing op-eds or otherwise conveying support for the witch hunt. Feminist icon and *Ms.* magazine co-founder Gloria Steinem is reported to have donated money to the McMartin investigation—specifically, efforts to dig up the grounds in search of secret tunnels.

In 1986, after three years of nationwide fury, prosecutors charged Buckey and six other McMartin employees with more than one hundred counts of child molestation and conspiracy, going to trial against him and his mother the following year, with a retrial of Buckey to follow in 1990. The press abetted prosecutors, vilifying the defendants and ignoring their counsel's statements. Journalist Geraldo Rivera aired a two-hour prime-time special, screened before church congregations, in which he alleged that at least one million people in the US were involved in a secretive criminal network of Satanists. Smith and Pazder also lent a hand, testifying for the prosecution. Still, there was not a single conviction in the case. Nor were there any findings of organized cult abuse at any other preschool or in the twelve-thousand-plus cases that had been alleged nationwide.

Though no one was convicted of organized ritual abuse, the Satanic Panic was a smashing victory for culture warriors. In the words of religion scholar Megan Goodwin, it effectively located the abuse of children "in the shadowy margins of American religion." It enabled the public to acknowledge the long-repressed fact of child sexual abuse while attributing it, as in past eras, to a monstrous, Christ-hating other. Some believers became so persuaded of evildoing on the part of Satanists that they viewed lack of evidence as *more* evidence—proof that their enemies were so "clever... eating those babies, bones and all."

Over the years, therapists would be exposed for planting false memories of satanic abuse in patients, undermining the credibility of their profession. MPD diagnoses would decline, as the scandal had cast doubt on the condition's legitimacy. (In 1994, the *DSM* renamed it dissociative identity disorder, also describing the condition as a splintering of identity, rather than the development of new personalities.) But the primary effects of the panic were even greater intolerance of minority religions and the continued abuse of children at the hands of clergy, scout leaders, relatives, and other familiar people. None other than Gothard victimized many, according to sources. The Basic Youth Conflicts founder resigned from his ministries in 2014, after thirty women alleged that he had molested or sexually harassed them or others in the workplace, some as minors. (An internal investigation found no criminal activity but acknowledged that Gothard had behaved "in an inappropriate manner.") Farris defended Gothard, and, citing parents' rights, his organization has continued to undercut legal safeguards for children, such as anonymous reporting.

Many child sex abuse victims of the '80s and '90s either attempted or died by suicide. David Cotton was among them. Feeling hopeless and unloved, he broke into a medicine cabinet at a group home and took handfuls of Thorazine and Tylenol. "I didn't think anyone cared about me," he says in retrospect. "I didn't want to live anymore." He was rendered unconscious before being given ipecac. After this incident, the courts got involved in his care. A judge wanted to institutionalize him. If it hadn't been for a social worker, he probably would have tried once more to end his life or found some equally tragic end. "That guy saved my life."

The social worker found David a foster family who lived on a forty-acre farm in the country. His foster parents weren't particularly kind, often calling him a dreamer and saying he would never amount to anything. But they mostly left him to his chores, which consisted of caring for the land and animals. More than seventy-five chickens roamed the place, along with cats, dogs, horses, and geese. He came to know the way ponds smelled after rain and the way the sun made shoots and twigs push up out of the earth. "For the first time, I was in a place that was God-made, not man-made, and that had an effect on me," he says. In that charged expanse, removed from human society, he began to feel that even in the midst of pain—*especially* in the midst of pain—he really wasn't alone. The God who had taken on broken, human flesh was with him, and whatever abuse he'd suffered need not be the last word.

His faith connected him to his mother, who, despite enduring her own hardships, had learned to take comfort in the being whose eye was always on the proverbial sparrow. And it helped him to show mercy toward his aunts. He came to think that, in contrast with his foster parents, Wilma and Helen might not have meant to hurt him. "Some people can't help what they do," he explains. "They were broken."

Besides directing the public eye away from incest and other mundane scenes of child abuse, the Satanic Panic shifted attention away from the social and psychological determinants of abuse.

Social reformers like Rush were drowned out by those who declared the devil to be responsible for children's wounds, also devoting resources to the prosecution of select suspects and the medicalization of abuse victims. By medicalizing victims, society made *patients* the problem to be fixed. And in further keeping with the neoliberal spirit of the day, professionals "fixed" such patients by encouraging them to draw upon their own inner strength to overcome ("get over") what had happened to them, a phenomenon well captured by the replacement of the term *victim* with the more heroism-forcing *survivor*. The question thus remained: Why do people hurt kids?

Among those who did want to understand sexual abuse, specifically in cases where the perpetrator had been victimized in childhood, Sándor Ferenczi's concept of "confusion of the tongues" remained compelling—or rather, was rediscovered. Jeffrey Moussaieff Masson's 1984 book *The Assault on Truth* revived Ferenczi's work in order to indict Freud for abandoning his seduction theory. The 1980s also saw the publication of psychoanalyst Leonard Shengold's *Soul Murder: The Effects of Childhood Abuse and Deprivation*, which argued that "the righteousness and religiosity" of abusive parents intensified the "compulsion to repeat." When parents presented themselves as godlike, abuse appeared to be "in consonance to the Order of the World" and the child was prone to submit, then later try to become like the righteous parent. Curiously, Shengold also identified in abuse victims a psychological obsession with rats and all they symbolized: animality, fecundity, dirt, disease, overconsumption, and, above all, biting. It was not unusual for victims to use their teeth on others, seeming to sense that they faced a choice: to bite or to be bitten. One cannot help but think here of Carl Morlok. But if child sex abuse contributed to the constable's oddities, this part of the story has been lost to history.

The Polish Swiss psychoanalyst Alice Miller suggested that spanking, which she deemed a form of sexual abuse, especially on the naked butt, increased the risk of antisocial behaviors in adulthood. Being spanked instilled the desire to inflict upon others the same pain and humiliation that were experienced at the hands of one's parents. Far from taming beasts, then, physical punishment *bred* them. Of course, the vast majority of spanked children did not grow up to abuse, just as the vast majority of child sex abuse victims did not grow up to abuse. Both were far more likely to be abused again as adults than they were to hurt others. It could be that, even as they were molesting David, Wilma and Helen were being victimized at the facilities they frequented. In the 1980s, investigative reporters with the *Detroit News* found that rape and mistreatment of patients were common at Northville State Hospital. Budget cuts, combined with high doses of psychiatric drugs, made it easy for staff and even other patients to assault those in care.

With the flourishing of trauma studies at the turn of the century, related theories have since developed to explain intergenerational abuse. Some experts allege that when sexual abuse occurs early in life, the child's feelings of shame and anger become entangled with their perception of sexual feelings, inclining the adult survivor to be aroused by assaultive scenes. In other words, the taboo aspects of the new abuse scene tap into memories and feelings of intimacy associated with an earlier one. Other experts offer that abuse victims simply may not recognize a healthy relationship, never having experienced one. (Wilma and Helen's most "normal" romantic relationships were with an older man and other hospital patients.) Still others suggest that survivors may be trying to undo their own abuse by reliving the relationship and reclaiming power. In the words of psychologist Elizabeth Hartney, they want to "get it right this time."

Though experts may disagree about what primarily underlies a predilection for child abuse, many are in consensus about the need for therapy to work through psychic conflicts, for the sake of both the individual and future generations. Even in the majority of cases where abuse victims do not grow up to physically harm young people, their trauma can be passed down.

But there would be no psychotherapy for Wilma and Helen. Not even after they endured another tragedy: their mother's death in 1983. An ever-changing drug regimen would be all.

The eighty-four-year-old Sadie died of cancer, reportedly telling her fifty-three-year-old daughters before she went, "You girls go on. Take care of yourselves and the house and live good Christian lives." After burying her, Sarah and Edna briefly vied against each other to lead the family. But the now-orphans couldn't manage long without their mother to negotiate between them and otherwise keep peace. Wilma moved into a halfway house, while Edna and Helen found an apartment supervised by state mental health social services. Sarah got the family home, which she shared with her older son until 1988, when it became too much to manage and a neighbor offered to buy it for $25,000 (about $64,000 today). He intended to demolish it to make a parking lot for his classic cars. David, who had just aged out of foster care, remembers his grandfather Carl's relatives showing up out of nowhere to pick the house clean. Long-lost brothers and cousins came and carried off oak tables, china hutches, guns, and family heirlooms brought from Germany. David made a point to at least get his grandfather's service revolver for himself. His mother only seemed to worry about preserving the silver bracelets that she and her sisters had worn at four years old.

The sale of the family home supplemented income that the quadruplets received from social service agencies, the licensing of their photograph to publishers of scientific textbooks, and the local community. After all these years, the quadruplets still had a few benefactors in town. Perhaps these charitable people sensed that they had their troubles, even though the newspapers had never printed a word about them. The press coverage, now infrequent, mostly told of the hobbies that kept the quadruplets busy in their golden years and their birthday celebrations, which provided an occasion for reporters to reflect on their dramatic entry into the world all those years ago.

There's little known about the next few decades of the quadruplets' lives with the noteworthy exceptions of the second follow-up study at NIMH and before that, an even greater loss for Sarah: the death of her older son in 1994. As David was then in a better phase of life, married and employed, he was able to help her through the crisis.

In the late 1980s, Bill had begun working for a carnival company. As a "carnie," he traveled surrounding states, helping to set up and break down equipment. One night, a tractor trailer severed his finger, and it took two hours to get to the nearest hospital. By the time he arrived, he required two quarts of blood. Not long after the transfusion, he became very sick and was diagnosed with HIV. The story was that the blood supply was tainted.

David and his mother tried to save Bill. David would go to the public library to search the web for any news of a cure. The federal government had initially been ungenerous with funding for cure research, with President Reagan going four years without acknowledging the epidemic. Activists and the media forced officials' hands eventually, including by turning an Indiana boy with hemophilia into the poster child of the disease. (Thirteen-year-old Ryan White was "an innocent victim of AIDS," as he had acquired HIV from a transfusion of infected blood, rather than sex or intravenous drug use.) Now that public and private drug researchers had more federal dollars, the words on many lips were "any day now."

What David most remembers about those years is the way his mother cared for his brother, especially toward the end. "She just didn't care if she got sick." She would hug him, mop his brow, sweep him off the bed, and carry him to the toilet or wherever else he needed to go.

Bill was only thirty years old when he died. He was buried in Chapel Hill Memorial Gardens, where his maternal grandparents rested. Dozens came to mourn the man who, after his taxi shift, would drive the highway looking for people who needed emergency roadside assistance. He'd even had business cards printed so no one would ever be stranded.

Years later, David admits he sometimes questions the story of the tainted blood supply. "The dates made sense, but was it the real truth? I didn't know. Could he have gotten it from somewhere else? Yes. Sometimes we have skeletons in the closet that we never talk about." But he also knows that, having endured sexual abuse, he can't trust his perception. It could very well be because *he* has secrets that he wonders about his brother.

It is common for sexual abuse survivors to project their own experience onto others or even onto new events in their own lives in the hope that the changed perspective will yield insights into what happened to them. Psychotherapist Galit Atlas writes that an abused child will revisit his traumatic experience at every developmental stage—when he becomes a teenager, when he has sex for the first time, when he has children, when his child reaches the age when the abuse occurred. "Time will not necessarily make the memory fade; instead, the memory will appear and reappear in different forms." Freud had a term for this process: *nachträglichkeit*, meaning "afterwardness." Though identified prior to abandoning his seduction theory, the concept appeared throughout his work, as he never denied that child abuse occurred in Victorian society, nor that it could come back to haunt a person long after the fact.

Was it also projection that made David think of sexual sin when his mother would become psychotic, screaming that she was going to hell? "She seemed to feel so guilty, and I just didn't know what else would make her feel that way." For many years, he made a point to keep pastors from visiting her. "I tried to keep them away or at the very least explain her severe anxiety and mental illness, so no talk about heaven or hell or doomsday talk. It's when they'd get on those subjects that I always had to pick up the aftermath."

He has never read *The Genain Quadruplets*, which describes Carl constantly threatening Sarah with damnation, offering another possible explanation of his mother's panic. For many years, the volume sat on the shelf in the Morlok family home, and he believed it to be about a different set of sisters studied at NIMH. Only recently did he learn that *Genain* was a pseudonym for his mother and aunts, and he hasn't since felt compelled to read what the scientists had to say about them. He remembers David Rosenthal as a kind man, but he never cared for Allan Mirsky. As he told Mirsky himself, he believed no good would ever come to his mother or aunts from their involvement with NIMH.

David said this in 1996, when the government researchers formally studied the quadruplets a third time. A chromosomal abnormality had just been found in Swedish triplets with schizophrenia diagnoses, and they were keen to know if the quadruplets bore the same abnormality. While they were at it, they could readminister neuropsychological tests, such as the continuous performance test, measuring sustained and selective attention in continuous tasks. By this point, the sisters were too aged to make the trip east, and so the scientists came to Lansing and set up shop at a nursing facility in town. Wilma was now residing in a home for the elderly with diagnoses of dementia and chronic obstructive pulmonary disease. Helen and Edna still shared an apartment together, while Sarah lived in her own home, renting out rooms to tenants. Helen was in slightly better health, and Edna and Sarah struck investigators as being in "fair" and "good" health, respectively. Helen, Wilma, and Edna were still taking decades-old antipsychotics, while Sarah had switched to risperidone, one of the many second-generation anti-psychotics touted to improve upon its predecessors, despite causing weight gain and high blood sugar.

Researchers conducted only brief interviews to determine recent health history. There were no psychotherapists to discern what occupied their conscious or unconscious minds.

The chromosomal oddity wasn't seen. Wilma's dementia was so bad that she could not understand basic commands or meaningfully participate in the neuropsychological tests. However, the other three did fairly well. In a 2000 paper appearing in *Schizophrenia Bulletin*, Mirsky compared the sisters' test scores at ages twenty-seven, fifty-one, and sixty-six, observing that each sister's cognitive performance either remained stable or improved. On this basis, he advanced the view that schizophrenia was a brain disease, though not necessarily a degenerative one as was commonly believed.

For all his emphasis on biology, Mirsky did continue to allow for the possibility that the sisters' life experiences had contributed to their outcomes—something that other renowned schizophrenia experts were now unwilling to do. After reviewing the study, the psychiatrist E. Fuller Torrey disagreed that psychosocial trauma such as the quadruplets had suffered was a contributing factor in schizophrenia. "There is no data to support that at all, except on a theoretical basis," said Torrey. Whatever unknown factor had interacted with genes to produce disease was "almost certainly biological," likely some sort of insult before birth. NIMH chief of neuropsychiatry Richard Wyatt agreed, specifically citing evidence of infection in the second trimester of pregnancy. Such comments betray the disparate burden of proof that had come to be required of psychosocial versus biological explanations. Without a complete laying bare of the way trauma changed the brain to produce psychosis, trauma could be written off as a "theoretical" cause of illness. Yet unspecific biological events authorized language like "almost certainly."

Mirsky's research team pressed David for a blood sample. He did give his arm, but only on three conditions: They test for HIV exposure, pay him several hundred dollars, and report any significant findings. He refused to participate in any neuropsychological tests and forbade researchers from taking a drop from his son, who had been born the year before. In his paper, Mirsky noted that David "was generally suspicious and mistrustful." Perhaps to further placate him as much as to recognize the quadruplets' contributions to scientific research, Mirsky's team paid the sisters a collective stipend of $1,000 (about $1,900 today). According to David, a representative of NIMH did report the negative result of the HIV screening, but not any other data. This seemed to indicate they'd found nothing of note, though, he'd later learn, unnamed NIMH researchers had already gone and told *Science* magazine that he was likely pre-schizophrenic. They cited his bad behavior in his youth.

It wouldn't be long before the first sister exited this world, followed by another, and then another. For all they'd offered of themselves, the genetics of schizophrenia remained unestablished. But just as this research door was closing, another much bigger one was opening. With the launch of the worldwide Human Genome Project, scientists looked to molecular genetics to find their smoking gun.

Chapter Sixteen

The Human Genome Project (1990–2003) brought together scientists from around the world to sequence the first human genome. In the United States, lead researchers included molecular biologist and geneticist James Watson, who, along with Francis Crick, discovered the structure of DNA, and biomedical scientist Charles DeLisi, then-spouse of Lynn DeLisi, who had authored several of the follow-up papers on the quadruplets. Estimated to take fifteen years and cost the US Department of Energy and the National Institutes of Health $3 billion, the project wrapped up two years early and slightly under budget.

Early in the project, researchers managed to map the inheritance pattern for Alzheimer's disease using a technique called linkage analysis, which compares the DNA of families affected by a disease to look for genetic markers that tend to be inherited together (that are "linked" during meiosis). Their success gave schizophrenia researchers great cause for hope. But in linkage studies of families affected by schizophrenia, positive findings were difficult to obtain and could not be replicated, prompting researchers to turn to the candidate gene approach. Here, researchers used a case-control study design to explore if potentially susceptible genes were associated with the disorder. Hundreds of candidate genes were tested, and some genes were identified as having "small effect" alleles (mutated forms with a very trivial link to schizophrenia). On the whole, however, the findings were underwhelming.

Next came the genome-wide association studies (GWAS), still popularly used. Rather than looking at a few genetic markers in certain loci, these studies allow for a comparison of genomes between populations with and without a given diagnosis. The rationale is that variants more common to the index group may be indicative of a genetic association. GWAS have identified 108 new susceptibility loci of very small individual effects, such as at dopamine receptor D2, in genes engaged in glutamatergic neurotransmission and synaptic plasticity, and in tissues implicated in core immune functions—findings believed to give credence to the hypothesized link between schizophrenia and dopamine and immune dysregulation, respectively.

Because none of these genetic variants can be considered causal, researchers have composed a polygenic risk score, which adds up all schizophrenia-associated variants in order to predict one's risk of developing the disorder. At present, polygenic score cards only explain about 3 percent of the variance in schizophrenic risk. By contrast, non-genetic factors explain about 17 percent of variance. Within this proportion, social factors, including migration and perceived status gap, account for 30 percent; environmental factors like childhood trauma account for 22 percent; and family history accounts for 24 percent. Though it is believed that polygenic score cards will become more predictive as GWAS sample sizes grow, some question how actionable these score cards will be, especially when a metric like family history—measuring relatives' psychiatric histories—already exists.

If the mapping of the human genome revealed how naive it was to suppose there might be a single gene behind schizophrenia, it also illuminated the complexity of gene-environment or epigenetic mechanisms. Epigenetic mechanisms include the process by which social or external stressors regulate the way the epigenome—a layer surrounding DNA—reads genes, as well as the process by which such modifications to the epigenome are passed down to future generations. The first is known as direct epigenetics and the second, indirect epigenetics. A direct epigenetic mechanism believed relevant to schizophrenia is methylation, whereby methyl groups join a molecule and repress gene transcription. Some researchers theorize that stress can modify DNA methylation, affecting the cells of people predisposed to develop schizophrenia and possibly erasing the evidence of involved genes. This modification to the epigenome can then be transmitted to descendants. When this happens, the basic sequence of DNA is unchanged; only the layer of instructions lying atop the DNA is imprinted by the parent's environment.

Epigenetics gained worldwide attention in 2015 when researchers claimed to have found a different chemical coating on the genes of children of Holocaust survivors—a seeming biological memory of what had happened to their parents. Researchers theorized that epigenomic modifications could influence how individuals respond to stress, disposing some to psychopathology. But some believe the investigators failed to isolate social and genetic factors and that such is impossible to do. In the words of one of the study's participants, "How does one separate the impact of horrific stories heard in childhood from the influence of epigenetics?"

When it comes to schizophrenia, clinical psychologist Jay Joseph sees the turn toward epigenetics and more sophisticated biological markers as an indication that research into biological origins is "reaching the desperation stage." Joseph has compared the pivot to methylation to the US government's actions following 9/11. At first, the government claimed it was sure to find weapons of mass destruction in Iraq. When that didn't happen, officials alleged the weapons had been destroyed or cleverly hidden. For psychologist Sharna Olfman, it's the "preformationist" bias of epigenetics talk that is problematic. Researchers acknowledge the role of epigenetic events but hold on to the notion of an "executive genome." They claim, for instance, that particular genomic variants are predisposed to epigenetic alterations, which then increase one's risk of schizophrenia diagnosis. "This perspective once again puts the cart (gene) before the horse (environment)," contributing to a "whack-a-mole" trend, whereby every time the latest notion of pre-formed personhood gets crushed, "a new version pops up to replace it."

It's not difficult to understand Joseph and Olfman's skepticism. The follow-up quadruplet studies and the commentary they engendered illuminate experts' relentless efforts to attribute serious mental illness to *some* primordial factor. The recent return of the notion that race is genetic—something firmly disavowed in the wake of the Holocaust—only further goes to show how junk science dies hard. But some believe it is critiques like Joseph's and Olfman's that are reflexive. In a piece titled "The Degenerative Agenda of Explaining Away Genetic Research in Schizophrenia," which specifically names Joseph, psychiatrist Awais Aftab notes that there is now wide consensus that schizophrenia is a complex trait, resulting from both genetic and environmental influences. "This is a pluralistic account," writes Aftab. "For all this rhetoric of reductionism directed at a pluralistic position, one has to wonder who is really being reductionistic here?"

The degenerative agenda that Aftab names may be nowhere more visible than in two critical descriptions of David Rosenthal, whose Danish-American studies with Seymour Kety and Paul Wender remain widely credited for offering some of the most convincing evidence of the genetic basis of schizophrenia to date. Beyond documenting the studies' flaws, psychiatrist Peter Breggin and clinical psychologist Richard Bentall have portrayed him as a zealot who maniacally pushed his genetics theory both in these studies and in *The Genain Quadruplets*. These portrayals reveal how roundly the sisters were exploited before any of their deaths. Similar to the way Freud engaged Daniel Paul Schreber's memoir while declaring real-life schizophrenics to be therapeutically hopeless, individuals of every theoretical persuasion treated their case as a text to be endlessly analyzed and interpreted—all while the four women lacked the chance to utter the word *I*.

In his 1991 book *Toxic Psychiatry*, written on the heels of the Satanic Panic, Breggin stated that Rosenthal's suggestion of a genetic etiology in the sisters' case was "a form of child abuse." Explaining how Rosenthal's book scatters mentions of abuse throughout the six hundred pages without ever analyzing its psychological impact, Breggin wrote, "To fail to underscore or to summarize the outrages perpetrated against the children constitutes intellectual complicity with the child abuser." In his 2003 book *Madness Explained*, Bentall similarly accused Rosenthal and his contributors of being so dogmatic—so "exclusively genetic"—that they shrugged off all the harms the sisters had suffered.

To say that the book pushed a singularly hereditarian view, Bentall and Breggin were obliged to ignore that the majority of *The Genain Quadruplets*' contributors were social workers, sociologists, and psychologists who could hardly be described as indifferent to environment. These experts scrupulously analyzed familial relationships, communication styles, and inner conflicts. While their inattention to abuse—or worse, recasting abuse in terms of timeless psychic traumas—was surely a shortcoming of the book, it is not evidence that they were gunning for genetics.

The sketch of Rosenthal as an extremist flew in the face of other facts. To start, Rosenthal admitted that it was self-serving for him and his colleagues to modify diagnostic criteria in the adoption studies. (And if he'd lived long enough, he'd have seen validation of the spectrum: Many psychiatrists now understand schizophrenia to exist on a continuum, with the difference between normal and abnormal being one of degree, rather than kind.) Second, he repeatedly urged that environment mattered, also recognizing that hallucinations were phenomenologically meaningful. Finally, there was the fact that the quadruplets and Sarah's living son were all very fond of Rosenthal. Were these people, all so deeply sensitive to harm, too stupid to intuit he was merely exploiting their tragedy to advance his career?

It's possible that Breggin and Bentall were reacting to the prejudice of medical textbooks, which Breggin rightly noted "grossly oversold [the Danish-American studies] to the profession and to the public." But should Rosenthal be pilloried for over-the-top appraisals of his work? It's not unthinkable a man as shy and modest as he would be surprised, perhaps even embarrassed, by the summaries, had he ever encountered them. More to the point, what good did it do the Morlok quadruplets—or any other child abuse victims—to describe one's ideological enemy as an abuser?

Now in his eighties, Breggin warns of "America-hating" globalists like George Soros, who desire to usher in a "new world order" by any means necessary, including the rampant harm of children through Covid-19 vaccination. Styled the "conscience of psychiatry," he also decries as "child abuse" the use of psychoactive medication in children with diagnoses like ADHD. Rosenthal, for his part, never gave up on the quadruplets, replying to their heart-rending letters, taking Edna's frantic phone calls, and continuing to travel to Lansing until he was forced to retire. Contrary to Bentall and Breggin's caricatures, he had the rare ability to let go of his own ambitions long enough to allow the quadruplets to speak. Perhaps it's this fact that ought to be remembered about him, especially as his successors at NIMH attempt to reimagine public psychiatry in the twenty-first century. Faced with the reality that the Human Genome Project and other billion-dollar research ventures haven't improved outcomes for those with serious mental illness, many in power have begun to ask who exactly NIMH is for—and how it might recommit to the humanitarian vision of its founders.

One of Rosenthal's final recorded visits to Michigan with Olive Quinn is particularly illustrative of his willingness to talk *with* them and not merely *about* them. Recounted in a 1977 publication, this visit is all the more curious for hinting at what is too often absent from the study and care of those with mental illness: a sense of professionals' own frailty, both unto themselves and in the faces of those who depend upon them.

By the time Rosenthal made this trip, his mind had begun to go. (Though he was the lead author on the essay bylined with Quinn, it's questionable if he meaningfully contributed to the writing.) He and Quinn had taken the family out to dinner when Edna began to hallucinate different figures, such as a man in a white coat. Quinn asked Edna to acknowledge that she was hallucinating, quoting George Herbert Mead on the nature of reality. When Edna could not disavow the man, instead appearing to listen to him, Quinn grew frustrated. She kept raising questions about the man's reality until Edna finally stated that he'd gone away, only now there was an examination bed in his place. If this bed was real, Quinn retorted, then Edna should go lie down in it. And once she did so, Quinn would be right behind her. The proposition seemed to confuse and embarrass Edna, and so Rosenthal made a joke to put her at ease. Finally, her eyes lit up and her face showed relief. The bed had disappeared.

Toward the end of the meal, she became distressed again. She claimed to feel very shaky and went to the bathroom. When she returned, she was still visibly uncomfortable. Something possessed Rosenthal to stand and guide her outdoors, where he took her hand and they walked together. Feeling that her palm was sweaty and trembling, he tried to reassure her that everything would be all right. He couldn't quite reach her, at least not to his satisfaction. But after a good night's sleep, Edna went three weeks without being bothered by any hallucinations—an unusually long reprieve, according to her mother.

There is something about this scene, the two of them each carrying burdens for which there were no words. Rosenthal regretted that he could not totally alleviate Edna's burden, but it's hard to imagine he didn't at least lighten it. Did she also lighten his? As someone who had repeatedly confronted death and come through the other side, she could relate to him in a way that few others could.

With their hunger for life, did the quadruplets ever stir feelings in other NIMH researchers, even if science's one-way gaze didn't allow for such sentiments to become part of the record? In the archives of the government institute, there sit boxes of data from blood tests, brain scans, skin tests, and psychiatric evaluations. There is little to document the pulled heartstrings, the moments of surprise or admiration, the realizations that these individuals had a point, that what they said made a strange sort of sense. And yet, it is not hard to imagine there *were* often pangs of feeling, even obligation, toward the women whom society had so horrifically failed. There *was* the knowledge, however fleeting, that in these women's cries for help, one had just heard an immemorial call for justice—a call to build for them the world they deserved and that NIMH was intended to bring about.

The brainchild of Robert Felix had begun as an attempt at the impossible, in that sense transcending politics. After fighting fascism abroad, the young military psychiatrist and his peers dreamed up a project radically opposed to the psychiatric establishment in Nazi Germany, where psychiatry had served as an agent of the authoritarian state. Psychiatry as they envisioned it would leverage the power of the government to usher in a world so wondrous that few would have cause to find themselves distressed. NIMH administrator Matthew Dumont captured this utopianism as late as 1968, five years following Kennedy's signing of the Community Mental Health Act. "The treatment of the ailing organism," he wrote, referring to the American city, "involves a redistribution of wealth and resources in this country on a scale that has never been imagined. We should be constructing a society for the urban poor of such beauty and richness, with so many options of behavior, that it becomes nothing less than a privilege to be called poor."

The notion that the last should be first had roots in many sacred texts, but it was a hard sell in post–civil rights America. Too many people preferred to bankrupt the federal government to avoid having to share any communal goods with the newly enfranchised; and NIMH soon abandoned social psychiatry for brain research. Americans with serious mental illness now help to compose the ranks of the "living dead," their outcomes considerably worse than those of their counterparts from previous decades and in other developed nations. Despite this fact, the government institute has remained committed to what is disparagingly referred to as the "bio-bio-bio model." And within white-dominated psychoanalytic circles, the Freudian doctrine of neutrality persists.

But there are some in high places who have permitted themselves to be interrupted, either by the cries of those who are hurting or by their own whims to forge a better way. Take Thomas

Insel, MD, who directed NIMH from 2002 to 2015, aggressively pushing for research into the genetics and neuroscience of mental illness. During his last year as the "nation's psychiatrist," Insel was delivering a PowerPoint on the latest findings on the genetic markers of schizophrenia when a man in the audience, who identified himself as the father of a twenty-three-year-old schizophrenic son, protested, "Our house is on fire, and you are talking about the chemistry of the paint. What are you doing to put out this fire?" In that moment, the psychiatrist was transformed. "I knew he was right," Insel writes in his 2022 memoir. "Nothing my colleagues and I were doing addressed the ever-increasing urgency or magnitude of the suffering millions of Americans were living through—and dying from." In fact, as the government was investing billions into the brain sciences, outcomes for those with serious mental illness were severely worsening. This was in no small part, he now knows, because "health is more about your zip code than your DNA code" and material conditions have only grown more dire for so many with mental illness. An entire generation was essentially left "to languish on our streets . . . eating out of trash bins."

While Insel is still hopeful for a day when brain research delivers a return for the public, and while he recognizes the failures of deinstitutionalization, he believes the time has come for NIMH to recommit to the ideals that inspired the Community Mental Health Act. In his words, "Kennedy's call to action and caring should still be our lodestar." In recent years, the federal government has taken some steps to rebuild the community care landscape, such as by funding sixty-six clinics in eight states to support those with mental illness or substance abuse. In contrast with the original Community Mental Health Centers, these Certified Community Behavioral Health Clinics offer crisis services, home visits, peer training, and outreach to homes, schools, and jails. They are paid prospectively—that is, for the population served, rather than time spent on services. This allows clinics to invest in the kinds of programs that prevent crisis. Many public health officials hope to see the centers expanded to other states.

Some psychoanalysts are also coming to grips with their complicity in perpetuating a psychologically destructive world, though not without pushback from within and beyond their own circles. The Jewish analyst Donald Moss found himself in hot water following the publication of an abstract for a forthcoming paper in which he defined "whiteness" as a malignant, parasitic-like condition characterized by "voracious, insatiable, and perverse" appetites directed at nonwhite people and their allies, necessitating psychic and social-historical interventions. According to Moss, psychoanalysts have largely failed to recognize whiteness, which primarily, but not exclusively, affects individuals with white skin.

Tucker Carlson and the far right pounced upon the abstract to make a case for white victimhood, many threatening death over social media or through the mail. Despite that those coming for the psychoanalyst with pitchforks and racist slurs ("filthy Jew") were vividly illustrating his hypothesis, many of Moss's peers stayed mum until the panic died down, then expressed regret that he had violated the profession's apolitical tradition with his "woke" screed. According to Hannah Zeavin, who wrote about the debacle involving Moss (her stepfather) for *n+1*, he was by no means the first to make "race and racism a central node of the psyche." Black psychoanalysts and thinkers had been doing so for some time. One could say this "lineage of thought was apparent even in Freud, who belonged to a marginalized category that marked him forever as the father of the 'Jewish Science.'" What distinguished Moss was that he was deemed a race traitor. He had exposed that which, in the words of scholar George Lipsitz, "never has to speak its name, never has to acknowledge its role as an organizing principle in social and cultural relations."

But there was one conference crowd that greeted Moss with a standing ovation; and prominent psychoanalyst Dorothy Holmes urged that readers give his paper a fair shake when it appeared in the *Journal of the American Psychoanalytic Association* (*JAPA*), alongside one she authored. These sympathetic minds appeared to understand that the analyst can never really coat-check social realities, if for no other reason than that thing Freud called the unconscious—and whiteness, for all its pretensions not to exist, was a social reality.

Beyond psychoanalytic circles, some are increasingly considering the physical and psychological effects of religious beliefs and practices, especially those that implicitly promote white racial dominance. According to psychotherapist Laura Anderson, who, along with licensed clinical social worker Brian Peck, co-founded the Religious Trauma Institute, both the Christian Nationalist iconography on display at the January 6 insurrection and the increased visibility of individuals exposing harm within religious spaces have led many to realize that high-control religion can get under the skin, giving rise to flashbacks, nightmares, nausea, hyperarousal, guilt, shame, dissociation, suicidal ideations, and more.

Anderson and Peck have coined the term *adverse religious experience* to refer to a religious experience that has not necessarily resulted in trauma, but that has been identified as a risk factor for trauma. One example that is particularly reminiscent of the quadruplets is having grown up in "purity culture," a modern chastity movement inspired by James Dobson's ministry wherein many teenage girls, typically evangelical or Catholic, pledge their premarital virginity to their fathers, wear silver rings to symbolize the covenant, and attend purity balls with Dad. Beyond having overtly incestuous themes, purity culture is accused even by theological conservatives of reducing young women's entire personhood to their sexuality and promoting a culture of rape. Much like under Carl Morlok's roof, virtues like honesty, charity, and kindness are little emphasized—the integrity of the hymen is all. And those who fail to adhere to strict dress codes, such as by letting their shoulders show or even wearing pants, are said to have "asked for" any sexual assaults they endure.

Many who were hyper-sexualized through purity culture have been diagnosed with PTSD, obsessive-compulsive disorder, bipolar disorder, borderline personality disorder, depression, anxiety, a food consumption disorder, or a dissociative disorder like schizophrenia, although Anderson questions if their symptoms might, at least in some cases, better approximate religious trauma. Religious trauma is, for her, a variant of the more recognized "complex trauma," which refers to trauma pursuant to prolonged or repeated events, such as child abuse or neglect.

Much skepticism surrounds the so-called semantic creep that has both professionals and members of the public scrutinizing religious upbringing and other common life experiences as a source of trauma. A *New York Times* headline conveyed this when it posed the question, "If Everything is 'Trauma,' Is Anything?" But as the author of that piece conceded, "Many things are genuinely not good" for Americans living today. And as Aftab noted in a Twitter thread on the medicalization of the term, "One could say that it is only by defining 'trauma' so broadly and loosely that [people] are able to see it everywhere."

The promise of trauma frameworks is, then, that they do not simply deal with the aftermath of violence, as do the conventional psychoanalytic space, drug therapy, and the *DSM*. They do not pretend all that matters is the psychic action in the room or the activity within the brain or the symptoms exhibited. They attend to societal violence and not in a way that romanticizes or minimizes individual disability. For these reasons, a growing number of psychiatrists and psychologists have begun to incorporate trauma-informed approaches into their practice. Many claim to have lost faith in the *DSM*, using its diagnostic codes purely for insurance reimbursement or professional advancement, such as when applying for grants or tenure, or when publishing in medical journals. Some align with the global Hearing Voices movement, which rejects that voices themselves are problematic, instead deeming one's relationship with those voices to be the source of distress. In Hearing Voices spheres, treatment is geared toward helping people learn to live with or control the voices in their heads, often by bearing witness to the trauma that those voices bespeak.

One can only wonder how the quadruplets might have benefited from people to help them recognize their terror of a God who so closely resembled their father, watching like a voyeur and then raining down wrath upon those who did not bend to his every maniacal whim. The way, in order to please this father-God, some of them became obsessed with contamination—with the filthy and the diseased and the forsaken. Yet trauma therapy, religious or otherwise, is not always more effective or humane than other forms of care. Sometimes in such a setting, trauma is the only thing people see; the other parts of a person are ignored or explained away as the mere products of trauma. Sometimes the question "What happened to you?" morphs into a violent command: "Show me your pain!" Sometimes individuals who desire medication or a more conventional diagnosis are told these wouldn't be helpful to them.

Today only one quadruplet survives, and she dispels any notion that her and her sisters' lives were singularly tragic. So do those who knew the family. Nearly one hundred years after their momentous births, Edna, Wilma, Sarah, and Helen live on in many more hearts than textbooks; and to those who remember them, they are testaments to the deep bonds of sisterhood and the power of hope, not any theory of mental illness. Denied love in childhood, they gave it to one another. Treated later in life like they belonged at the bottom of society, they knew they were actually precious. Endlessly given reasons to despair, they kept believing in better things to come.

Chapter Seventeen

Sometimes when their father was not home, the quadruplets stole away to a frozen pond to skate. They were only eight or nine years old then. Carl had never permitted them to buy ice skates, claiming they were too expensive. And so it was in their shoes that they tried to glide across the surface. They surely made for an awkward sight, pulling one another and trying to turn figure eights only to collapse on the ice. Yet it was only bliss they would remember about those days.

Even though they feared their father from the time they were in cribs, there were many times, over the years, that the four sisters defied him. When Carl tried to sabotage their education, sending them to bed before they could finish their homework, they began to sneak their books to their rooms. They'd pretend to fall asleep and then turn on the light after they could hear his snoring. They took pride in their accomplishments, and they were not going to let him get in their way.

When Carl forbade them from leaving the house, they transformed the house to resemble other settings. "We would move the dining chairs to the living room, so it looked like school or church," Sarah once reminisced. "If it was church, Edna or I would play hymns on the piano, and the other one of us would give a sermon. Then Wilma and Helen would come up for communion." Shortly before Carl was expected home, they'd scramble to replace the furniture. Their mother never let on about their play.

Mental illness surely devastated their lives, and, at different times, took each of them to very dark places. But it did not extinguish the fires inside. Well into her golden years, Wilma refined her skills as a hair and makeup artist, and composed hundreds of poems, which she enclosed in holiday cards to friends and relatives. Helen never held down a job, but she also wrote her own poems and even prayers, which she would recite. The more she aged, the more she came to take interest in both the services and community at Emanuel First Lutheran Church. She kept a list of all the friends she made there and would read it to herself, savoring just how many people had come to love her. Edna and Sarah worked as secretaries, also learning to play 265 hymns and songs by ear on the organ or piano. Helen so delighted in all of the sisters' talents that she often wrote to apprise movie stars of their goings-on, signing her letters "The Morlok Quadruplets."

Even more stirring than their accomplishments, though, is the way they bore one another up and out of every valley. Many who studied them in Bethesda viewed their intimacy purely as a psychic catastrophe. By identifying with one another, these experts said, they mimicked one another's pain and distress. Were it not for their "poor ego boundaries," they might have fared better. But wasn't it also by seeing and being seen that they knew they were never alone?

If Carl's hate was too easily flattened to pathology, so, it seems, was the sisters' love. The likes of Olive Quinn idealized an individuated self—a self that could distinguish itself from others, that came into being by knowing exactly where it ended and another began.

But the subjectivity that the quadruplets embodied was much more undone. In the figure of Wilma begging to stay home from school with Helen, one sees a self that is ready to bleed for another. In the figure of Sarah staying under the family roof to prevent Carl from punishing the others, a self that is willing not to individuate. And in the figures of Helen telling NIMH staff to "give Wilma the pill" and Edna taking Sarah's baby for walks even though it pained her, selves that choose compassion over their own survival.

This kind of love exceeded the tools that the researchers had at their disposal. It sometimes seemed to sneak up on one or another of them, as when a therapist noted that perhaps Helen's gobbledygook was actually the "language of the heart." But they could not cut it down to size and hold it up to the light. In that way, at least, it *was* like madness, only ever flashing its face—or one of them—before slipping away.

Wilma was the first to go. In January 2002, she was admitted to Sparrow Hospital with pneumonia, dying only a few hours later. The seventy-one-year-old was honored with a memorial service at Emanuel First Lutheran and then buried in Chapel Hill Memorial Gardens, where her sisters took a long walk and shared memories. None of them ever wanted to forget the way she'd tell a joke and then slap her knee before anyone got the punch line. Nor even the way she went about all her business with a cigarette dangling from her lips. They agreed her chain-smoking had probably contributed to her death.

The following year, Helen died at her home of unspecified causes. As Sarah was out of town and she was so distraught, Edna had to call the police, who sent a female officer to comfort her. Among Helen's belongings was a stash of literature from the Salesian

Missions, a Catholic missionary organization that she'd apparently been supporting for years. Who knew what it was about this particular charity, outside her own tradition, that sparked something in her? Perhaps, in the faces of the world's poor, she saw herself and wanted to instill hope the way that she thought best: by letting the dispossessed know they were deeply, unreservedly loved by God.

After her death, Edna decided to telephone one of the boys who'd been mean to Helen in grade school. She wanted him to say sorry for what he'd done. "I was just a kid," the now-old man replied. But seeing Edna meant business, he offered an apology, along with his condolences.

Edna and Sarah then grew closer. The longtime "frenemies" moved into the same apartment building, taking daily walks and getting together for bingo and other amusements. On her own, Sarah began to make scrapbooks of known sets of twins, triplets, quadruplets, and quintuplets. All her life, she'd felt connected to other multiples, as if they were all part of some mystical circle—a communion of saints, but for people who'd shared their first, watery home. This work led her to research her own family, and before long, she found herself writing a book about herself and her sisters.

In 2007, Edna moved to foster care. It had become too difficult for her to manage on her own. Three years later, the two surviving quadruplets celebrated their eightieth birthday by going out to dinner and then visiting Sparrow Hospital to see a special exhibit. Employees had put together a big display of artifacts from their childhood, including their Raggedy Ann and Andy dolls, favorite books, and recital dresses. The following year, Edna was transferred to a health care facility. Sarah regularly visited, and one day while doing so, the both of them were surprised by a visit from Dr. Allan Mirsky. He'd come all the way to Michigan with a few student interns, who looked them up and down and then administered two diagnostic tests, one to evaluate their ability to shift attention and another to assess their ability to focus on a task. For old times' sake, the two surviving sisters sang "Alice Blue Gown," nearly bringing Mirsky to tears. Sarah wrote about this visit in her memoir, published in 2015, the same year that Edna died and two years after Mirsky et al. published a letter to the editor of *Schizophrenia Research* hailing antipsychotics and unspecified community support for helping the quadruplets to lead relatively normal lives.

The Morlok Quadruplets, by Sarah Morlok Cotton, did not delve into the details of their abuse, although it did portray Carl as domineering and even violent at times. "We really were like little tin soldiers with tunnel vision, and we marched to every beat," wrote Sarah, adding that Carl was "just plain possessive... he really thought he could prevent [his children] from growing up." She explained how Carl especially loathed his youngest. If Helen was ever too slow to answer a question at the dinner table, he would lean over the table and smack her with a knife. Sarah and Edna had to change seats so she would be out of his reach. "As we grew older," she went on, "we realized our father was a real tyrant and ridiculed us a lot and made us feel worthless, which gave us low esteem. We were like birds in a gilded cage." These words marked the first time she had publicly acknowledged things weren't as blissful as outsiders perceived. It must have taken great courage for her to put them on the page.

In a chapter on their years at NIMH, Sarah reinforced the idea that the family had gone to be studied as multiples. She claims not to be secretive about mental illness—she just prefers to focus on what makes her proud. These days, she loves to read well-wishes from multiples around the world, as well as to peruse her archive of family memorabilia. She has amassed all kinds of relics that she won't permit anyone to throw away: graduation programs, artwork that her sons drew in elementary school, and locks of their hair. She now lives in a small adult foster care home in Plymouth, between Lansing and Detroit. Her son David regularly visits and brings her to his home for dinners with her grandchildren. She also keeps in touch with two cousins on her mother's side, who describe her as loving and joyful. She takes a handful of psychoactive drugs. These seem to prevent acute psychosis, even if they have side effects. It has been years since she's had a bad episode.

Sarah credits her faith for helping her out of the darkness of her childhood. Like her sister Helen, she has learned to take comfort in her own prayers and devotions. Even if there are moments when the past overtakes her, her Bible is no longer bookmarked to passages describing the apocalypse, but instead to the poetry of an oppressed people come upon green pastures and still waters. She has found her way, both literally and figuratively, from the Book of Revelation to the Book of Psalms. The God of her favorite psalm is not a vengeful one, but a shepherd whose rod and staff comfort. Not an enemy who desires her suffering, but a friend who prepares tables and makes cups runneth over.

After several decades of estrangement, her son has recently decided to meet with his father, now eighty-six and still living in Florida. "Maybe I can get answers," says David. "Maybe I can find out what happened to make him the way he was." Sarah is very curious to know what he uncovers. In recent days, she has begun to realize how much she never knew about her own parents, especially her father. It was plain that Germany was his castle in the sky, but beyond that, she heard very little about his boyhood.

There are some mysteries that will always surround Carl—and thus, the quadruplets—no matter what scientists discover about the human brain or genome. When and how exactly did Old

World passions pack themselves into his little body, and what if he'd realized how much they wore him down? Had Carl looked hard at himself in the mirror, would he still have tossed at night, or would he have been able to love his children, to laugh with them instead of at them? Would there have been ice skates and friends and light coming through the windows at the house on East Saginaw Street?

If there is one truth to which the quadruplets' lives attest, it is that there *are* consequences of burying history. But there is also, always, the possibility of reparation. What happened cannot be undone, but it is also not destiny. If the ghosts of the past haunt the living—and they always do, in one form or another—there is power in naming them. And having named them, working toward a world where all people share in the wealth of the earth and there is no hunger, no hate, and no children who tremble.

Author's Note

This work of nonfiction synthesizes material from David Rosenthal's 1963 book *The Genain Quadruplets*; his war diary and private letters; Sarah Morlok Cotton's 2015 memoir *The Morlok Quadruplets*; the quadruplets' diaries, letters, and effects; scientific and scholarly publications; newspaper articles; medical records; and interviews with Cotton, her son David, Rosenthal's three children, and others with knowledge of the Morlok family or NIMH studies. With such an array of perspectives, some discrepancies were noted, mostly pertaining to dates. In these situations, I relied on my intuition. All the recounted events and quotations are factual, though some quoted material has been edited for clarity and grammar, and many quotations reflect individuals' memories of dialogue occurring years or even decades prior. Some events have been omitted at Sarah's request. With the exceptions of the quadruplets' classmate "Sally Murphy," Northville patients "Thomas" and "Lenny," and the Morloks' neighbor "Mrs. Wheeler," whose real names could not be confirmed, no pseudonyms have been used. Loretta is Sarah's best recollection of the name of her paternal uncle Bill's wife.

I have taken the liberty of narrating individuals' feelings and reactions in more descriptive terms. If, for instance, a source described someone as embarrassed, I might write that her face turned red. For the sake of pacing, I have also rendered certain scenes—notably, those set at NIH's Clinical Center—in real time when they are based on source material published several years after the fact. Because the quadruplets stayed at the center from 1955 to 1958, some years before the release of Rosenthal's book, it is possible that certain contributors' insights were more retrospective than suggested here. I have, however, made an effort to avoid chronological errors, such as by confirming that theories described in the 1963 book had been introduced by the mid-1950s. All scientific and scholarly citations can be found in the endnotes.

Acknowledgments

Girls and Their Monsters began with a phone call from my mother. While reading Robert Kolker's *Hidden Valley Road*, she had come across a fascinating story within the story: Four quadruplets had all been diagnosed with schizophrenia following a traumatic childhood. It was a strange case of nature versus nurture, and it could be my next book. After hanging up, I googled the Genain quadruplets and found Patrick Hahn's essay on them in *Mad in America*. I was intrigued enough to spend $300 on Rosenthal's now-out-of-print book, a few pages into which I knew that my mother had been right. Thank you, Mom, and also Bob and Patrick, for dropping these first bread crumbs.

The central argument of this book—that long before the Morlok quadruplets became the poster children of psychiatric genetics, they were the poster children of an unacknowledged but potent mythology—was not exactly an easy one to articulate in the early stages of book plotting. It began as a series of hunches—that this or that detail might mean more than met the eye, that so and so might have more to say. My agent Marya Spence had enough confidence in the story to take its loose ends to Maddie Caldwell and her assistant Jacqui Young, who immediately saw the potential and who quickly came to love Edna, Wilma, Sarah, and Helen. What an honor to bring a second book into the world with these three brilliant women. Many thanks, as well, to Mackenzie Williams of Janklow & Nesbit, and to the rest of the Grand Central Publishing team: publicist Roxanne Jones, marketer Alana Spendley, cover designer Sarah Congdon, copyeditor Laura Jorstad, and production editor Bob Castillo.

I'm grateful for my independent fact checker Andy Young, who carefully reviewed the scientific and historical material. Some parts were tweaked after he did his bit, and I accept full responsibility for any errors.

A lot of smart people patiently answered research questions or pointed me toward other experts and resources. My heartfelt gratitude to author Susannah Cahalan, sociologist Andrew Scull, and psychiatrist Awais Aftab for their knowledge on the history and philosophy of psychiatry. Thanks to neuropsychologist Allan Mirsky, evolutionary psychologist and behavioral geneticist Nancy Segal, clinical psychologist Jay Joseph, and author Catherine Rakow for their comments on the quadruplets' case. Mirsky needs no introduction. Segal worked as Rosenthal's assistant in the 1970s and has written extensively about twins. Joseph has published various critical accounts of the quadruplet studies, and Rakow is an expert on the life and work of Murray Bowen, the psychiatrist who ran the ward where the Morloks initially stayed at the Clinical Center. All of their perspectives were invaluable.

So were those of Evelyn Beck and Joyce Griffin, the maternal cousins of the quadruplets, and Suellen Hozman, Bill Cotton's AIDS buddy. Hozman founded the Lansing Area AIDS Network, getting to know Bill and his relatives as part of her work for that charity. These three attested to the incredible love and kindness of the Cotton family, even in times of tragedy.

I am indebted, as well, to Joel Pless, dean of the Wisconsin Evangelical Lutheran Synod Seminary, for answering my questions about divorce in the 1920s, and Maria Erling of the United Lutheran Seminary for identifying Pless as the right person to field those queries. Psychotherapist Laura Anderson kindly sat for an interview about religious trauma, while religion scholar and founder of the After Purity Project Sara Moslener let me pick her brain about purity culture. While writing this book, I was fortunate to participate in a Moslener-led *Straight White American Jesus* seminar on race, sex, and disembodiment.

Though I did not explicitly cite it in the preceding pages, I have been greatly influenced by Christian psychologist Richard Beck's *Unclean: Meditations on Purity, Hospitality, and Mortality*, which considers how theological calls to sanctity lure the faithful into practices of social exclusion, even genocide. Also deserving of mention: Candida Moss's *The Myth of Persecution: How Early Christians Invented a Story of Martyrdom*, which considers how false and highly stylized tales of predatory others have long galvanized the church.

The archivists who graciously gave their time, in some cases providing scanned materials, include Heidi Butler of the Capital Area District Libraries; Ashley Washington and Daishyana Banks of NIH's Clinical Center; and John Rees of the National Library of Medicine. Ian Rosenthal, nephew of the late David, kindly gave permission for me to reproduce photographs taken by his father, Arthur.

My friends Kate Sprague, Katy Giebenhain, and Lizzie Berne DeGear encouraged me with their ongoing interest in this story, and the whip-smart Brigid Duffy read and commented on early drafts. Brigid let me know which paths to abandon and which to wander down, also sprinkling her magic dust on many of the sentences.

Thanks go to Jason Linkins, who gave me opportunities to share facets of my research for the *New Republic*. Like others named here, Jason has a knack for seeing a story even when I have only the germs of an idea.

This book would not be the same without the generosity of Rosenthal's surviving children. Scott and I met for many cups of coffee, and Laura once joined the two of us for lunch. Amy and I were able to speak by phone. Within the first minutes of conversation with Scott, I realized that the psychologist at the heart of this narrative was so much larger than I had fathomed—and thus, that I had an enormous responsibility in bringing him to life on the page. In the end, Rosenthal's persona shaped the arguments of the book, not just the plot. Where I had initially been tempted to join the crowds calling to burn down the psychiatric establishment, his compassion toward the quadruplets persuaded me that reform could—and always has—come from within.

There is another David who lights up these pages, and that is David Cotton. He could have ignored my Facebook message, but instead welcomed me into his life and shared his story. Hearing of his deep love for his mother, I rested assured that this quadruplet really had gotten her happy ending. And it was because of him that I came to know and love this woman, too.

Sarah, what to say? When David gave me your number, I never expected you to return my call, but you did. For every question I asked, you had one of your own, saying in your folksy way, "I'm as interested in *you* as you are in *me*." Before long, we'd exhausted our memories of the past, and so the phone calls became about the present: what the Rosenthal children were up to, my son's baseball slump, the drama at your retirement home. After you prayed for Henry to get a hit, I put the phone on speaker so you could hear the crack of the bat—and there was one! Then there was the time you tried to say goodbye so you could sneak to the kitchen with your walker for a forbidden dessert. "Just put me on hold," I said, anxious to know how your plan unfolded. A few minutes passed, and then I heard "I'm baaaack." We laughed so hard that I worried the aide was going to find you out.

Being with you in person has been even more memorable. I think of the way you always scoot closer to me on the couch, putting your hand on my knee. And the time David was going on about pulverized metals and I turned to whisper in your ear, "You are *such* a gift." Your eyes twinkled, and you replied, "I know." Sarah, thank you for all the ways you've enriched my life and for trusting me to tell this story, which I dedicate to you.

Endnotes

PROLOGUE

4 **the estimated frequency:** Rosenthal, David (1963). "Introduction." In *The Genain Quadruplets: A Case Study and Theoretical Analysis of Heredity and Environment in Schizophrenia.* Ed. David Rosenthal. New York: Basic Books, p 5.

CHAPTER ONE

8 **Freud described:** "The Primal Scene: What Did the Interpretation of the Wolf Man's Dream Reveal?" Freud Museum. 2018. https://www.freud.org.uk/education/resources/the-wolf-mans-dream/the-primal-scene/. Retrieved October 3, 2022.

13 **While Michigan law:** Laws Relating to the Registration of Births, Deaths and Marriages; the Licensing and Solemnizing of Marriages, and Laws Concerning Divorce. State of Michigan. Revision of 1925, p 25. Available here: https://www.google.com/books/edition/Laws_Relating_to_the_Registration_of_Bir/xYNxAAAAIAAJ?hl=en&gbpv=1&printsec=frontcover. Retrieved October 3, 2022.

14 **The church was part:** Braun, Mark (2003). *A Tale of Two Synods: Events That Led to the Split Between Wisconsin and Missouri.* Pewaukee, WI: Northwestern Publishing, pp 43–44.

15 **Abortion was not officially outlawed:** An anti-abortion law took effect the following year. See the Michigan Penal Code, Act 328 of 1931. Available here: https://www.legislature.mi.gov/documents/mcl/pdf/mcl-328-1931-III.pdf. Retrieved October 3, 2022.

15 **but it was extremely dangerous:** Gold, Rachel Benson (2003). "Lessons from Before Roe: Will Past Be Prologue?" *Guttmacher Policy Review* 6.1. Available here: https://www.guttmacher.org/gpr/2003/03/lessons-roe-will-past-be-prologue. Retrieved October 3, 2022.

CHAPTER TWO

19 **A news writer remarked:** "Mr. Morlok's Calamity Turns Out an Unexpected Blessing" (June 22, 1930). *San Francisco Examiner*, p 81.

19 **Going back centuries:** Obladen, Michael (2021). "Unwelcome: The Abominable Twins." In *Oxford Textbook of the Newborn: A Cultural and Medical History*. Oxford, UK: Oxford University Press, pp 116–22.

19 **For much of human history:** Pentikäinen, Juha (1990). "Child Abandonment as an Indicator of Christianization in the Nordic Countries." *Scripta Instituti Donneriani Aboensis* 13, pp 72–74.

20 **Real and imagined loafers:** Wood, Dan, and Soren Jordan (2017). *Party Polarization in America: The War Over Two Social Contracts*. Cambridge, UK: Cambridge University Press, pp 94, 97–98.

20 **Michigander Henry Ford:** Ford, Henry. "Ford Lays Slump to Era of Laziness" (October 3, 1930). *New York Times*, p 7.

20 **In the early decades:** Raffel, Dawn (2019). *The Strange Case of Dr. Couney: How a Mysterious European Showman Saved Thousands of American Babies*. New York: Penguin Random House, p 68.

20 **A Chicago physician:** Dyrbye, Amy (n.d.). "The Black Stork." Eugenics Archive. https://eugenicsarchive.ca/discover/tree/517224eceed5c60000000012. Retrieved October 3, 2022.

21 **"Quadruplets Win Election for Daddy":** "Quadruplets Win Election for Daddy" (November 4, 1931). *Brooklyn Times Union*, p 4.

21 **The Lansing mayor:** Actual quote: "He could have run for US senate and been elected. He had no qualifications *whatever*" (emphasis added). Quoted in Perlin, Seymour (1963). "Anamnesis." In *The Genain Quadruplets: A Case Study and Theoretical Analysis of Heredity and Environment in Schizophrenia*. Ed. David Rosenthal. New York: Basic Books, p 53.

22 **Countless books have described:** See, for instance, Smith, Lillian (1949). *The Killers of the Dream*. New York: Norton; and Hernton, Calvin (1965). *Sex and Racism in America*. New York: Doubleday.

22 **statues only being:** Smith 121.

22 **Viewing Black women:** Hernton 95.

23 **the kidnapping of the beloved aviator's son:** Carolyn Cox (2021). *The Snatch Racket: The Kidnapping Epidemic That Terrorized 1930s America*. Sterling, VA: Potomac Books, jacket.

24 **This created many highly dramatized manhunts:** Kosner, Edward (February 25, 2021). "'The Snatch Racket' Review: Coppers & Kidnappers." *Wall Street Journal*. https://static1.squarespace.com/static/5f2c40760917a13cf69a52e6/t/603e35c8ce30b65195f5b477/1614689738503/Ed+Kosner+'The+Snatch+Racket'+Review_+Coppers+%26+Kidnappers+-+WSJ+%281%29.pdf. Retrieved October 3, 2022.

26 **Some parenting manuals urged:** Hawkes, Gail L., and Danielle Egan (December

2008). "Developing the Sexual Child." *Journal of Historical Sociology* 21.4, p 443.

26 **Believing that masturbation:** Schatzman, Morton (1973). *Soul Murder: Persecution in the Family.* New York: Random House, pp 99–100.

26 **including castration:** Schatzman 49–50.

26 **For German doctor:** Schatzman 37–41, 79.

28 **At the high-water mark:** "Fitter Family Contests." Eugenics Archive. http://www.eugenicsarchive.org/html/eugenics/static/themes/8.html. Retrieved October 3, 2022.

29 **Americans' fascination:** Lantz, Susan Jennings (2014). "America's Lollipop Licking Tease: The Eroticization of the Female Child in 1930s Film." PhD Dissertation, West Virginia University. Graduate Theses, Dissertations, and Problem Reports 461. https://researchrepository.wvu.edu/etd/461, pp 16–19.

29 **Even President Franklin Delano Roosevelt:** Lantz 55.

CHAPTER THREE

31 **It all started:** Miller, Sarah (2019). *The Miracle & Tragedy of the Dionne Quintuplets.* New York: Schwartz & Wade, pp 59–61.

31 **the Ontario government passed:** Walker, Melissa (November 4, 2019). "The Dionne Quints Were Premature and Tiny. But Fame Was the Real Problem." *New York Times.* https://www.nytimes.com/2019/11/04/books/review/the-miracle-and-tragedy-of-the-dionne-quintuplets-sarah-miller.html. Retrieved October 3, 2022.

31 **Three million people:** Miller 121.

32 **whose images were licensed:** Miller 127, 134; see also Brockell, Gillian (November 3, 2019). "The Dionne Quintuplets: The Exploitation of Five Girls Raised in a 'Baby Zoo.'" *Washington Post.* https://www.washingtonpost.com/history/2019/11/03/dionne-quintuplets-exploitation-five-girls-raised-baby-zoo/. Retrieved October 3, 2022.

32 **The proceeds from these ventures:** Brockell (November 3, 2019).

37 **Norman Rockwell was painting:** Halpern, Richard (2006). *Norman Rockwell: The Underside of Innocence.* Chicago: University of Chicago, pp 108, 112–13, plate 7.

37 **Morton's Salt Girl:** "Seasons of Change." Morton Salt. https://www.mortonsalt.com/heritage-era/seasons-of-change/. Retrieved October 3, 2022.

37 **The Tinseltown toddler:** Lantz, Susan Jennings (2014). "America's Lollipop Licking Tease: The Eroticization of the Female Child in 1930s Film." PhD Dissertation, West Virginia University. Graduate Theses, Dissertations, and Problem Reports 461. https://researchrepository.wvu.edu/etd/461, pp 48–50.

37 **she was a top-grossing:** "Shirley Temple Receives $50,000 per Film." History.com. https://www.history.com/this-day-in-history/shirley-temple-receives-50000-per-film. Retrieved October 3, 2022.

37 **including a Black man:** Lantz 65.

37 **In a review of *Wee Willie Winkie*:** Lantz 46.

37 **Indeed, J. Edgar Hoover:** Kasson, John F. (2014). *The Little Girl Who Fought the Great Depression: Shirley Temple and 1930s America.* New York: Norton, p 116.

37 **One studio executive unzipped:** Black, Shirley Temple (1988). *Child Star: An Autobiography.* New York: McGraw Hill, pp 319–20.

38 **Another used a remote switch:** Temple (1988) 431–32.

38 **A producer attempted to seduce her:** Temple (1988) 429.

38 **expressed outrage:** Kasson 81–82; see also Anderson, L. V. (February 12, 2014). "What Was the Deal with Graham Greene Calling Shirley Temple 'a Fancy Little Piece'?" *Slate.* https://slate.com/culture/2014/02/graham-greene-and-shirley-temple-what-to-make-of-the-novelists-sexual-review-of-wee-willie-winkie.html. Retrieved October 3, 2022.

38 **In the words of Susan Jennings Lantz:** Lantz 43.

38 **who wrote to Temple's producer:** Lantz 64.

39 **Drawing upon Freudian:** Karman, Benjamin (1951). "The Sexual Psychopath." *Journal of Criminal Law and Criminology* 42.2, pp 193, 197; see also Van De Water, Marjorie (October 10, 1937). "The Facts About Sex Crimes." *Oklahoma City News,* p 12; and Porter, Marion (September 5, 1937). "Wanted: A Law to Hold Sex Criminals." *Courier-Journal,* p 50.

39 **In the case of homosexuals:** Freedman, Estelle B. (June 1987). "Uncontrolled Desires: The Response to the Sexual Psychopath, 1920–1960." *Journal of American History* 74.1, p 89.

39 **Sexual psychopath laws:** Lave, Tamara Rice (2009). "Only Yesterday: The Rise and Fall of Twentieth Century Sexual Psychopath Laws." *Louisiana Law Review* 69, p 570.

39 **The Morloks' home state:** Lave 549, 571.

39 **In the words of Charles E. Morris, III:** Morris III, Charles E. (May 2002). "Pink Herring & The Fourth Persona: J. Edgar Hoover's Sex Crime Panic." *Quarterly Journal of Speech* 88.2, p 238.

40 **Across the nation:** Freedman 94.

40 **White psychiatry declared:** Summers, Martin (2019). *Madness in the City of Magnificent Intentions: A History of Race and Mental Illness in the Nation's Capital.* Oxford, UK: Oxford University Press, pp 81, 141.

40 **Popular culture promoted:** Pilgrim, David (2000). "The Brute Caricature." Jim Crow Museum. https://www.ferris.edu/HTMLS/news/jimcrow/brute/homepage.htm. Retrieved October 3, 2022.

40 **Griffith's 1915 film:** Rampell, Ed (March 3, 2015). "'The Birth of a Nation': The Most Racist Movie Ever Made." *Washington Post.* https://www.washingtonpost.com/posteverything/wp/2015/03/03/the-birth-of-a-nation/. Retrieved October 3, 2022.

40 **The blockbuster movie:** "Klansville: The Film Birth of a Nation Glorified the KKK." PBS. https://www.pbs.org/video/klansville-film-birth-nation-glorified-kkk/. Retrieved October 3, 2022.

40 **Klansmen and other racial terrorists:** "Lynching in America: Confronting the

Legacy of Racial Terror." Third edition. Equal Justice Initiative. https://lynchinginamerica.eji.org/report/. Retrieved October 3, 2022.

40 **these lynchings were not confined:** "Racial Terror Lynchings." Equal Justice Initiative. https://lynchinginamerica.eji.org/explore. Retrieved October 3, 2022.

40 **Following the separate murders:** Robertson, Stephen (2006). *Crimes Against Children: Sexual Violence and Legal Culture in New York City, 1880–1960.* Chapel Hill and London: University of North Carolina Press, p 155; see also French, Mary (May 22, 2018). "At Einer Sporrer's Grave." New York City Cemetery Project. https://nycemetery.wordpress.com/2018/05/22/at-einer-sporrers-grave/. Retrieved October 3, 2022.

43 **the police had refused to investigate:** "Malcolm X: Formative Years in Michigan" (2022). Michigan State Archives. https://michiganology.org/stories/malcolm-x-formative-years-in-michigan/. Retrieved October 3, 2022.

44 **dying later at Sparrow Hospital:** Russell, Jessica (2020). *The Life of Louise Norton Little: An Extraordinary Woman: Mother of Malcolm X and His 7 Siblings* (e-book), p 183.

44 **They provided "a kind of looking glass":** Quinn, Olive W. (1963). "The Public Perception of the Family." In *The Genain Quadruplets: A Case Study and Theoretical Analysis of Heredity and Environment in Schizophrenia.* Ed. David Rosenthal. New York: Basic Books, p 371.

CHAPTER FOUR

47 **President Roosevelt signed into law:** "President Roosevelt Signs Selective Training and Service Act." History Unfolded: US Newspapers and the Holocaust. https://newspapers.ushmm.org/events/president-roosevelt-signs-selective-training-and-service-act. Retrieved October 3, 2022.

50 **Psychoanalysis dominated:** Harrington, Anne (2019). *Mind Fixers: Psychiatry's Troubled Search for the Biology of Mental Illness.* New York: Norton, p 82.

50 **When Clark University:** Skues, Richard (2012). "Clark Revisited: Reappraising Freud in America." In *After Freud Left: A Century of Psychoanalysis in America.* Ed. John Burnham. Chicago: University of Chicago Press, pp 56–57.

50 **In a series of lectures:** Freud, Sigmund (April 1910). "About Psychoanalysis." *American Journal of Psychology* 21. Reprint: https://www.rasch.org/over.htm. Retrieved October 3, 2022.

50 **It was the first time:** Burnham, John (2012). "Introduction." In *After Freud Left: A Century of Psychoanalysis in America.* Ed. John Burnham. Chicago: University of Chicago Press, p 14.

51 **made an immediate impression:** Matthews, F. H. (1967). "The Americanization of Sigmund Freud: Adaptations of Psychoanalysis Before 1917." *Journal of American Studies* 1.1, p 40.

51 **While some did indeed rebuff:** Harrington (2019) 37.

51 **Advertisers soon began:** Samuel, Lawrence R. (2010). *Freud on Madison Avenue:*

Motivation Research and Subliminal Advertising in America. Philadelphia: University of Pennsylvania Press; see also Held, Lisa (December 2009). "Psychoanalysis Shapes Consumer Culture." *Monitor on Psychology* 40.11, https://www.apa.org/monitor/2009/12/consumer. Retrieved on October 3, 2022.

51 **For those who couldn't afford:** Matthews 41; see also "Freud and Freudianism" (October 27, 1924). *TIME.* https://content.time.com/time/subscriber/article/0,33009,719355,00.html; and "Medicine: Intellectual Provocateur" (June 26, 1939). *TIME.* https://content.time.com/time/subscriber/article/0,33009,931342,00.html. Retrieved October 3, 2022.

51 **bestsellers like Dr. Benjamin Spock's:** Hidalgo, Louise (August 23, 2011). "Dr. Spock's Baby and Child Care at 65." BBC. https://www.bbc.com/news/world-us-canada-14534094. Retrieved October 3, 2022.

51 **If by midcentury:** Harrington (2019) 80.

51 **At a time when journalists:** Harrington (2019) 109–10.

52 **By some accounts:** Parsons, William B. (2021). *Freud and Religion: Advancing the Dialogue.* Cambridge, UK, and New York: Cambridge University Press, p 40; see also Ignatieff, Michael (June 12, 1986). "The Jewish Freud." *New York Review of Books.* https://www.nybooks.com/articles/1986/06/12/the-jewish-freud/. Retrieved October 3, 2022.

52 **the Roman Catholic Church:** Lavin, Talia (September 29, 2020). "QAnon, Blood Libel, and the Satanic Panic." *New Republic.* https://newrepublic.com/article/159529/qanon-blood-libel-satanic-panic. Retrieved October 3, 2022; see also Szasz, Thomas (1978). "The Jewish Avenger." In *The Myth of Psychotherapy.* Syracuse, NY: Syracuse University Press, pp 138–58.

52 **Freud determined to replace:** Szasz 144.

53 **he developed a sixty-item rubric:** Rosenthal, David (1955). "Changes in Some Moral Values Following Psychotherapy." *Journal of Consulting Psychology* 19.6, pp 431–36.

54 **being reconceived:** Harrington (2019) 96.

54 **Both the nineteenth-century:** Heckers, Stephan (November 2011). "Bleuler and the Neurobiology of Schizophrenia." *Schizophrenia Bulletin* 37.6, pp 1131–35.

54 **saw a few studies:** Johnson, Josephine (September 2013). "The Ghost of the Schizophrenogenic Mother." *Journal of Ethics.* https://journalofethics.ama-assn.org/article/ghost-schizophrenogenic-mother/2013-09. Retrieved October 3, 2022; see also Harrington, Anne (2016). "Mother Love and Mental Illness: An Emotional History." *History of Science and the Emotions* 31.1, pp 106–07.

54 **In 1940:** Fromm-Reichmann, Frieda (1940). "Notes on the Mother Role in the Family Group." *Bulletin of the Menninger Clinic* 4.5, pp 132–48; see also Harrington (2016) 106.

54 **Here Fromm-Reichmann suggested:** Fromm-Reichman, Frieda (1948). "Notes on the Development of Treatment of Schizophrenics by Psychoanalytic Psychotherapy." *Psychiatry* 11.3, pp 263–73.

54 **researchers sought to prove:** Harrington (2019) 95.

55 **Fromm-Reichmann believed even the most disturbed:** Harrington (2019) 97; and Harrington (2016) 107.

55 **was planning to investigate:** Parloff, Morris (2002 B). Interview by Ingrid Farreras. Office of NIH History and Stetten Museum. https://history.nih.gov/display/history/Parloff%2C+Morris+2002+B. Retrieved October 3, 2022.

55 **Twin studies had long been cited:** Kety, Seymour S. (1995). Interview by Irwin J. Kopin. Office of NIH History and Stetten Museum. https://history.nih.gov/display/history/Kety%2C+Seymour+S.+1995. Retrieved October 3, 2022.

56 **psychiatrist Ernst Rüdin and his mentee Franz Josef Kallmann:** Kurbegovic, Erna (September 13, 2013). "Ernst Rudin." Eugenics Archive. http://eugenicsarchive.ca/discover/tree/5232a9bb5c2ec50000000023. Retrieved October 3, 2022; Benbassat, Carlos A. (April 2016). "Kallmann Syndrome: Eugenics and the Man Behind the Eponym." *Rambam Maimonides Medical Journal* 7.2. https://www.ncbi.nlm.nih.gov/pmc/articles/PMC4839542/. Retrieved October 3, 2022; and Benbassat, Carlos A. (April 2016). "Kallmann Syndrome: Eugenics and the Man Behind the Eponym." *Rambam Maimonides Medical Journal* 7.2. https://www.ncbi.nlm.nih.gov/pmc/articles/PMC4839542/. Retrieved on October 3, 2022.

56 **was unpopular to think:** Kety, Seymour S. (1996). "Seymour S. Kety." In *The History of Neuroscience in Autobiography*, volume 1. Ed. Larry R. Squire. Washington, DC: Society for Neuroscience, p 402; see also Stahnisch, D. (September 13, 2013). "Twin Studies." Eugenics Archive. http://eugenicsarchive.ca/discover/tree/5233682e5c2ec5000000003e. Retrieved October 3, 2022.

56 **He was certain:** Kety, Seymour S. (1995, 1996).

56 **The newly formed institute:** Farreras, Ingrid, Caroline Hannaway, and Victoria A. Harden, eds. (2004). *Mind, Brain, Body, and Behavior: The Foundations of Neuroscience and Behavioral Research at the National Institutes of Health.* Biomedical and Health Research series 62. Amsterdam: IOS Press, p 7.

56 **At a time:** Farreras, Hannaway, and Harden xiv.

56 **The National Mental Health Act of 1946:** Farreras, Hannaway, and Harden 60.

57 **a research psychologist named Morris Parloff:** Parloff (2002 B).

CHAPTER FIVE

61 **giving credence:** Foucault, Michel (1978). *The History of Sexuality*, volume 1. Trans. Robert Hurley. New York: Pantheon, p 21. Available here: http://www.freudians.org/wp-content/uploads/2014/09/The-History-of-Sexuality-1-Michel-Foucault-The-History-of-Sexuality-Volume-1_-An-Introduction-Pantheon-Books-1978.pdf. Retrieved October 3, 2022.

61 **The father of psychoanalysis:** Robinson, Paul (1993). "Jeffrey Masson: Freud, Seduction, and the New Puritanism." *Freud and His Critics.* Berkeley: University of California Press, pp 101–78.

62 **"great clinical secret":** Freud, Sigmund (October 15, 1895). Letter to Wilhelm

Fliess. In *The Complete Letters of Sigmund Freud to Wilhelm Fliess, 1887–1904*. Psychoanalytic Electronic Publishing. Available here: https://pep-web.org/search/document/ZBK.042.0144A. Retrieved October 3, 2022.

62 **he adopted the motto:** Fletcher, John (2013). *Freud and the Scene of Trauma*. Baltimore: Johns Hopkins University Press, p 4.

62 **A growing discourse:** Harrington, Anne (2019). *Mind Fixers: Psychiatry's Troubled Search for the Biology of Mental Illness*. New York: Norton, pp 93–94.

66 **German psychiatrist Richard Freiherr von Krafft-Ebing:** Oosterhuis, Harry (April 2012). "Sexual Modernity in the Works of Richard von Krafft-Ebing and Albert Moll." *Medical History* 56.2, pp 133–55.

66 **Michigan physician and eugenicist:** Saha, Joy (December 4, 1921). "Once a Cure for Deviant Behaviors, Kellogg's Corn Flakes Continue to Be a Blueprint for All Cereals." *Salon*. https://www.salon.com/2021/12/04/once-a-cure-for-deviant-behaviors-kelloggs-corn-flakes-are-blueprint-for-breakfast-cereals/. Retrieved October 3, 2022.

66 **Kellogg also blamed:** Kellogg, John Harvey (1881). *Plain Facts for Old and Young*. Burlington, IA: Segner & Condit. Republished by Project Gutenberg. https://www.gutenberg.org/files/19924/19924-h/19924-h.htm. Retrieved October 3, 2022.

66 **While formulating his seduction theory:** Makari, George J. (Winter 1998). "Between Seduction and Libido: Sigmund Freud's Masturbation Hypotheses and the Realignment of His Etiologic Thinking, 1897–1905." *Bulletin of the History of Medicine* 72.4, pp 647–49.

66 **Later accepting that infants:** Sauerteig, Lutz (April 2012). "Loss of Innocence: Albert Moll, Sigmund Freud and the Invention of Childhood Sexuality Around 1900." *Medical History* 56.2. Available here: https://www.ncbi.nlm.nih.gov/pmc/articles/PMC3381499/. Retrieved October 3, 2022.

68 **"doing their bit":** "Clean Plate Campaign Launched in Lansing" (July 25, 1943). *Lansing State Journal*, p 1.

69 **"In our city":** "Happy Birthday for 'Quads,' 13, Despite Gloom" (May 19, 1943). *Lansing State Journal*, p 1.

69 **as the *Lansing State Journal* did:** "Colorful Parade Here Is Seen by Thousands" (September 2, 1924). *Lansing State Journal*, p 7.

69 **One writer reported:** "Happy Birthday for 'Quads,' 13, Despite Gloom."

70 **"I hope nobody believes":** "Morlok Quads Unsteadily Observe Tenth Birthday" (May 18, 1940). *St. Joseph Herald-Press*, p 5.

70 **"Their pleasures and most of their fun":** "Michigan's Noted Morlok Quads Enter Their Teens" (May 16, 1943). *Detroit Free Press*, p 57.

70 **"In case you are under any misapprehensions":** Brown, Vivian (October 8, 1944). "Quad Quandary." *Lansing State Journal*, p 18.

71 **Lansing welfare workers:** Russell, Jessica (2020). *The Life of Louise Norton Little: An Extraordinary Woman: Mother of Malcolm X and His 7 Siblings* (e-book), p 3.

71 **welfare workers denied:** Russell 186.

71 **paid her a smaller stipend:** Russell 187.

71 **disapproved of her driving a car:** Russell 5–6.

71 **When she became pregnant:** Solomon, Jolie (March 21, 2022). "Overlooked No More: Louise Little, Activist and Mother of Malcolm X." *New York Times.* https://www.nytimes.com/2022/03/19/obituaries/louise-little-overlooked.html. Retrieved October 3, 2022.

71 **one of whom had been caught:** Russell 251.

71 **A physician diagnosed:** Russell 239.

71 **Around their birthday:** "Michigan Quadruplets Enter Their Teens" (May 13, 1943). *Detroit Free Press*, p 1.

71 **In the pursuant story:** "Michigan's Noted Morlok Quads Enter Their Teens" (May 16, 1943). *Detroit Free Press*, p 57.

72 **an *Escanaba Daily Press* writer imagined:** "Lansing Quads Have Birthday" (May 20, 1943). *Escanaba Daily Press*, p 1.

CHAPTER SIX

73 **Nor did the two scientists:** Gardner, Iva C., and H. H. Newman (September 1943). "Studies of Quadruplets: V—The Only Living One-Egg Quadruplets." *Journal of Heredity* 34.9, pp 259–63.

79 **This was the attitude:** Huber, Valerie J., and Michael W. Firmin (Winter 2014). "A History of Sex Education in the United States Since 1900." *International Journal of Educational Reform* 23.1, p 36.

79 **Advocates countered:** Huber and Firmin 30–33.

79 **Thanks to the influence of racial purists:** Slominski, Kristy (February 2021). "Medical Men, Moralists, and the Roots of Sex Education." *Teaching Moral Sex: A History of Religion and Sex Education in the United States.* Oxford, UK: Oxford University Press, pp 19–66.

86 **This characterization stemmed:** Metzl, Jonathan (2010). *The Protest Psychosis: How Schizophrenia Became a Black Disease.* Boston: Beacon, pp 38–39.

86 **Only four years later:** Metzl 82.

CHAPTER SEVEN

95 **a drug injected:** "Shock Therapy." Restoring Perspective: Life and Treatment at the London Asylum. Western University Archives. https://www.lib.uwo.ca/archives/virtualexhibits/londonasylum/shock.html. Retrieved October 3, 2022.

95 **Patients compared:** Whitaker, Robert (2003). *Mad in America: Bad Science, Bad Medicine, and the Enduring Mistreatment of the Mentally Ill.* New York: Basic Books, p 95.

95 **the New York State Psychiatric Institute:** Whitaker 93.

95 **"The greater the damage":** Read, John (March 4, 2021). "Shocked." *Aeon.* https://aeon.co/essays/why-is-electroshock-therapy-still-a-mainstay-of-psychiatry. Retrieved October 3, 2022.

95 **performing Rosemary Kennedy's botched lobotomy:** Harrington, Anne (2019). *Mind Fixers: Psychiatry's Troubled Search for the Biology of Mental Illness.* New York: Norton, p 71.

98 **In his much-revered:** Bleuler, Eugen (1950). *Dementia Praecox, or the Group of Schizophrenias.* Trans. Joseph Zinkin. New York: International Universities Press, p 102. Available here: https://philarchive.org/archive/BLEDPO-2. Retrieved October 3, 2022.

98 **It didn't seem to cross Bleuler's mind:** van der Kolk, Bessell (2015). *The Body Keeps the Score: Brain, Mind, and Body in the Healing of Trauma.* New York: Penguin, p 25.

98 **Sigmund Freud was even more convinced:** Paul Ricoeur famously described Freud as having a "hermeneutics of suspicion." See his *Freud and Philosophy* (1977). Trans. Denis Savage. New Haven, CT: Yale University Press.

99 **revealed paranoid delusions:** Schatzman, Morton (1973). *Soul Murder: Persecution in the Family.* New York: Random House; and Niederland, William G. (1984). *The Schreber Case: Psychoanalytic Profile of a Paranoid Personality.* Oxfordshire, UK: Routledge.

99 **chalked the author's issues:** Freud, Sigmund (2003). *The Schreber Case.* Trans. Andrew Webber. New York: Penguin Random House.

99 **Nineteenth-century physician:** Cartwright, Samuel A. (1851). "Report on the Diseases and Physical Peculiarities of the Negro Race." *New Orleans Medical and Surgical Journal*, pp 691–715.

99 **whose confinement at Kalamazoo:** Tubbs, Anna Malaika (2021). *The Three Mothers: How the Mothers of Martin Luther King, Jr., Malcolm X, and James Baldwin Shaped a Nation.* New York: Flatiron, p 121.

99 **When asylums began:** Smith, Kylie M. (July 6, 2020). "Discrimination and Racism in the History of Health Care." National Alliance on Mental Illness. Available here: https://nami.org/Blogs/NAMI-Blog/July-2020/Discrimination-and-Racism-in-the-History-of-Mental-Health-Care. Retrieved October 3, 2022; and Summers, Martin (2019). *Madness in the City of Magnificent Intentions: A History of Race and Mental Illness in the Nation's Capital.* Oxford, UK: Oxford University Press, pp 5, 154–55.

99 **Such was the case:** Russell, Jessica (2020). *The Life of Louise Norton Little: An Extraordinary Woman: Mother of Malcolm X and His 7 Siblings* (e-book), p 5.

100 **medical doctors were actually beginning:** Beck, Richard (2015). *We Believe the Children: A Moral Panic in the 1980s.* New York: Public Affairs, pp 2–3.

100 **This was true:** Herman, Judith Lewis (1981). *Father-Daughter Incest.* Cambridge, MA: Harvard University Press, p 18.

100 **Kinsey's findings:** Herman 16.

101 **a French surgeon had accidentally found:** Ban, Thomas A. (August 2007). "Fifty Years Chlorpromazine: A Historical Perspective." *Neuropsychiatric Disease and Treatment* 3.4, pp 495–500; see also Harrington, *Mind Fixers,* 98–100.

102 **In 1952, the US pharmaceutical company:** Whitaker 150.

106 **the public had gone hysterical:** Driver, Justin. "Of Big Black Bucks and Golden-Haired Little Girls: How Fear of Interracial Sex Informed *Brown v. Board of Education* and Its Resistance." In *The Empire of Disgust: Prejudice, Discrimination, and Policy in India and the US*. Ed. Zoya Hasan et al. Oxford, UK: Oxford University Press, pp 41–61.

106 **knowing a ruling:** Nussbaum, Martha (2018). *The Monarchy of Fear: A Philosopher Looks at Our Political Crisis.* New York: Simon & Schuster Paperbacks, p 123.

CHAPTER EIGHT

109 **cornerstone laid by President Truman:** Lyons, Michelle (2015). "History Mystery Part 1: President Truman and the Clinical Center Cornerstone." Intramural Research Program Blog. National Institutes of Health. Available here: https://irp.nih.gov/blog/post/2015/06/history-mystery-part-1-president-truman-and-the-clinical-center-cornerstone. Retrieved on October 3, 2022.

109 **Lorraine-cross shape:** Farreras, Ingrid, Caroline Hannaway, and Victoria A. Harden, eds. (2004). *Mind, Brain, Body, and Behavior: The Foundations of Neuroscience and Behavioral Research at the National Institutes of Health.* Biomedical and Health Research 62. Amsterdam: IOS Press, p 64.

109 **If someone had:** Parloff, Morris (2002 B). Interview by Ingrid Farreras. Office of NIH History and Stetten Museum. https://history.nih.gov/display/history/Parloff%2C+Morris+2002+B. Retrieved October 3, 2022.

112 **Parloff found it so difficult:** Parloff (2002 B).

114 **Rosenthal was overwhelmed:** Rosenthal, David (1963). "Introduction." In *The Genain Quadruplets: A Case Study and Theoretical Analysis of Heredity and Environment in Schizophrenia*. Ed. David Rosenthal. New York: Basic Books, p 7.

114 **His mind turned to Bénédict Augustin:** Rosenthal, "Introduction," 5–6.

115 **The more Rosenthal came to know:** Rosenthal, "Introduction," 7.

115 **Their case was more useful:** Rosenthal, "Introduction," 5.

115 **some experts assumed:** Rosenthal, David (1963). "A Suggested Conceptual Framework." In *The Genain Quadruplets: A Case Study and Theoretical Analysis of Heredity and Environment in Schizophrenia*. Ed. David Rosenthal. New York: Basic Books, p 508.

115 **the constitutional predisposition could be:** Rosenthal, "Suggested Conceptual Framework," 507.

115 **there was disagreement:** Rosenthal, "Suggested Conceptual Framework," 541, 549.

CHAPTER NINE

119 **These two hatreds:** Egid, Jonathan (April 22, 2022). "Pseudoscience as Policy." *Times Literary Supplement.* https://www.the-tls.co.uk/articles/hybrid-hate-tudor-parfitt-book-review-jonathan-egid/. Retrieved on October 3, 2022.

119 **many experts had begun to wonder:** Thomas, Alexander, and Samuel Sillen (2000). *Racism and Psychiatry.* New York: Citadel, pp 106, 114–15.

119 **Or maybe infantile tendencies:** Sterba, R. (1947). "Some Psychological Factors in Negro Race Hatred and in Anti-Negro Riots." In *Psychoanalysis and the Social Sciences.* Ed. G. Róheim. New York: International Universities Press, pp 411–27.

120 **Wanting his program:** Zeavin, Hannah (Spring 2022). "Unfree Associations: Parasitic Whiteness On and Off the Couch." *n+1* 42. https://www.nplusonemag.com/issue-42/essays/unfree-associations/. Retrieved October 3, 2022.

120 **Hitler became known:** Thomas and Sillen 112–13.

120 **When Jewish analysts fled:** Zeavin.

121 **NIMH's ranks included no Black psychiatrists or psychologists:** Geller, Jeffrey (September 22, 2020). "Structural Racism in American Psychiatry and APA: Part 7." *Psychiatric News.* https://psychnews.psychiatryonline.org/doi/full/10.1176/appi.pn.2020.10a33.

121 **far less willing:** Zeavin.

121 **she presented the Morlok family:** Rosenthal, David (1963). "Psychiatric Disorders in the Families of Mr. and Mrs. Genain." In *The Genain Quadruplets: A Case Study and Theoretical Analysis of Heredity and Environment in Schizophrenia.* New York: Basic Books, p 176.

123 **His caseworker characterized:** Hirsch, Stanley I. (1963). "A Caseworker's View of Mr. Genain." In *The Genain Quadruplets: A Case Study and Theoretical Analysis of Heredity and Environment in Schizophrenia.* Ed. David Rosenthal. New York: Basic Books, p 441.

125 **"dominated by a selfish, irascible mother":** Hirsch 446.

125 **Electroencephalographic studies revealed:** Evarts, Edward V. (1963). "Electroencephalographic Studies of the Genain Family." In *The Genain Quadruplets: A Case Study and Theoretical Analysis of Heredity and Environment in Schizophrenia.* New York: Basic Books, pp 206–07; see also Rosenthal, David (1963). "Possible Inherited Factors: EEG Abnormality." In *The Genain Quadruplets: A Case Study and Theoretical Analysis of Heredity and Environment in Schizophrenia.* New York: Basic Books, p 514.

125 **both father and daughters:** Rosenthal, "Possible Inherited Factors: EEG Abnormality," 515, 532.

125 **Two experts further deduced:** Hutt, Max (1963). "Bender-Gestalt Test." In *The Genain Quadruplets: A Case Study and Theoretical Analysis of Heredity and Environment in Schizophrenia.* New York: Basic Books, p 253; see also Rosenthal, David (1963). "Possible Environmental Factors: Life-Experience." In *The Genain Quadruplets: A Case Study and Theoretical Analysis of Heredity and Environment in Schizophrenia.* New York: Basic Books, p 556.

126 **Sadie used all sorts:** Basamania, Betty W. (1963). "The Development of Schizophrenia in the Child in Relation to Unresolved Childhood Conflicts in the Mother." In *The Genain Quadruplets: A Case Study and Theoretical Analysis of Heredity and Environment in Schizophrenia.* New York: Basic Books, pp 450–51.

126 **"One can surmise":** Undated medical note. Patient files of Sadie Morlok. NIH Clinical Center. Reprinted with permission of Sarah Morlok Cotton.

127 **Sadie's caseworker described:** Basamania 449, 452–53.

127 **Sadie never had the chance:** Basamania 453.

127 **Sadie imparted:** Basamania 459.

128 **she treated each:** Basamania 465.

128 **Carl was almost entirely off the hook:** Basamania 466.

129 **declared Sadie to be:** Singer, Margaret Thaler (1963). "A Rorschach View of the Family." In *The Genain Quadruplets: A Case Study and Theoretical Analysis of Heredity and Environment in Schizophrenia*. New York: Basic Books, pp 317–18.

129 **also using speech:** Singer 316.

129 **For the test evaluator:** Singer 319.

129 **blindly evaluated:** Schaefer, Earl S. (1963). "Parent-Child Interactional Patterns and Parental Attitudes Toward Child-Rearing." In *The Genain Quadruplets: A Case Study and Theoretical Analysis of Heredity and Environment in Schizophrenia*. Ed. David Rosenthal. New York: Basic Books, p 424.

129 **a construct newly developed:** See Theodor W. Adorno et al. (1950). *The Authoritarian Personality.* New York: Harper & Brothers.

129 **The Morlok patriarch answered:** Schaefer 420–21.

129 **Attempting to make sense:** Schaefer 424.

130 **The founder himself:** Thomas and Sillen 120–21.

130 **It was utter defeatism:** Thomas and Sillen 106.

130 **They were bolstered by a flowering:** Sluzki, Carlos E. (2007). "Lyman C. Wynne and the Transformation of the Field of Family-and-Schizophrenia." *Family Process* 46.2, pp 143–49. Available here: https://sluzki.com/publications/articles/147/lyman-c-wynne-and-the-transformation-of-the-field-of-family-and-schizophrenia. Retrieved October 3, 2022.

131 **One in-house psychologist:** Mishne, Judith Marks (1993). *The Evolution and Application of Clinical Theory: Perspective from Four Psychologies.* New York: Free Press, p 101.

CHAPTER TEN

132 **Though doll play:** Rosenthal, David (1963). "Editor's Note." In *The Genain Quadruplets: A Case Study and Theoretical Analysis of Heredity and Environment in Schizophrenia*. Ed. David Rosenthal. New York: Basic Books, p 326.

135 **She was also struck:** Usdansky, Blanche Sweet. "Doll Play." In *The Genain Quadruplets: A Case Study and Theoretical Analysis of Heredity and Environment in Schizophrenia*. Ed. David Rosenthal. New York: Basic Books, p 331.

136 **Edna, Wilma, and Helen had their own:** Usdansky 339, 350.

136 **Edna struck:** Usdansky 344.

136 **Wilma was more animated:** Usdansky 338.

136 **Helen gave the impression:** Usdansky 344.

136 **Edna was more cooperative:** Kendig, Isabelle V. (1963). "The Draw-a-Person Test." In *The Genain Quadruplets: A Case Study and Theoretical Analysis of Heredity and Environment in Schizophrenia.* Ed. David Rosenthal. New York: Basic Books, p 257.

136 **Sarah's women were satisfactorily:** Kendig 263–64.

136 **Edna's women were stiff:** Kendig 259.

136 **Wilma's one woman:** Kendig 266.

137 **Helen was the only sister:** Kendig 268.

137 **Blindly analyzing Rorschach protocols:** Singer, Margaret Thaler (1963). "A Rorschach View of the Family." In *The Genain Quadruplets: A Case Study and Theoretical Analysis of Heredity and Environment in Schizophrenia.* Ed. David Rosenthal. New York: Basic Books, p 324.

137 **Sarah and Helen also identified:** Singer 324.

137 **Helen described hatchets:** Singer 323.

137 **Another psychologist who blindly evaluated:** Piotrowski, Zygmunt A. "Rorschach Diagnostic Evaluations." In *The Genain Quadruplets: A Case Study and Theoretical Analysis of Heredity and Environment in Schizophrenia.* Ed. David Rosenthal. New York: Basic Books, pp 279, 293–95.

137 **evaluated samples:** Rosenthal, David, and Thea Stein Lewinson. "Handwriting of the Quadruplets During Premorbid and Morbid Conditions." In *The Genain Quadruplets: A Case Study and Theoretical Analysis of Heredity and Environment in Schizophrenia.* Ed. David Rosenthal. New York: Basic Books, p 227.

137 **Lewinson also identified:** Rosenthal and Lewinson 233.

137 **Lewinson noted:** Rosenthal and Lewinson 233–34.

138 **Around twenty-five staff members recorded:** Schaefer, Earl S. (1963). "Parent-Child Interactional Patterns and Parental Attitudes Toward Child-Rearing." In *The Genain Quadruplets: A Case Study and Theoretical Analysis of Heredity and Environment in Schizophrenia.* Ed. David Rosenthal. New York: Basic Books, p 399.

138 **One, presumably a nurse, described:** Schaefer 415.

138 **The collected observations:** Schaefer 399.

138 **Rosenthal later explained:** Rosenthal, "Editor's Note," 269.

138 **a sociologist named Olive Quinn was studying:** Quinn, Olive W. "The Public Image of the Family." In *The Genain Quadruplets: A Case Study and Theoretical Analysis of Heredity and Environment in Schizophrenia.* Ed. David Rosenthal. New York: Basic Books, p 355.

139 **Lyman Wynne suspected:** Wynne, Lyman, et al. (September 1957). "Family Relations of a Set of Monozygotic Quadruplet Schizophrenics." International Congress of Psychiatry. Psychiatric Abstract Series 12. US Department of Health, Education, and Welfare. https://books.google.com/books?id=PWcIgoM90vkC&pg=PA70&lpg=PA70&dq=lyman+wynne+%22monozygotic+quadruplet%22&source=bl&ots=B8jyOcePif&sig=ACfU3U3HHrb4WqSF6asny0-BStHqbgPG1w&hl=en&sa=X&ved=2ahUKEwis8tOl9Ln5AhXDEGIAHSXpBJMQ6AF6BAgQEAM#v=onepage&q=lyman%20wynne%20%22monozygotic%20quadruplet%22&f=false. Retrieved October 3, 2022.

139 **The communications scholar Gregory Bateson:** Bateson, Gregory, et al. (1956). "Toward a Theory of Schizophrenia." *Behavioral Science* 1.4, pp 251–54. Available here: https://solutions-centre.org/pdf/TOWARD-A-THEORY-OF-SCHIZOPHRENIA-2.pdf. Retrieved October 3, 2022, p 4.

139 **Naturally the person became:** Bateson 6.

139 **whom Bateson et al. cited:** Bateson 16.

144 **After some psychiatrists:** McCarthy-Jones, Simon (2017). *Can't You Hear Them?: The Science and Significance of Hearing Voices.* London: Jessica Kingsley, p 212.

144 **the company had launched:** Harrington, Anne (2019). *Mind Fixers: Psychiatry's Troubled Search for the Biology of Mental Illness.* New York: Norton, pp 101–02.

CHAPTER ELEVEN

148 **had only praise for Carl:** "Quads Dad Dies at 68" (August 9, 1957). *Lansing State Journal*, p 1.

148 **Ferenczi believed:** Ferenczi, Sándor (1949). "Confusion of the Tongues Between the Adults and the Child." *International Journal of Psychoanalysis* 30, p 226.

148 **Anna Freud expounded:** Freud, Anna (1936). *The Ego and the Mechanisms of Defense.* London: Karnac Books, pp 109–21.

149 **According to Rosenthal and two colleagues:** Rosenthal, David, et al. (1963). "The NIH Years." In *The Genain Quadruplets: A Case Study and Theoretical Analysis of Heredity and Environment in Schizophrenia.* Ed. David Rosenthal. New York: Basic Books, p 153.

150 **Woodley House was designed:** Rothwell, Naomi, and Joan Doniger (1963). "Myra at Woodley House." In *The Genain Quadruplets: A Case Study and Theoretical Analysis of Heredity and Environment in Schizophrenia.* Ed. David Rosenthal. New York: Basic Books, p 161.

151 **The FDA had now approved:** Compazine was approved in 1956 and Trilafon in 1957. Scherer, Leo (November 30, 1957). "Tranquilizers Major Aid at State Hospitals Here, Doctors Believe." *Lincoln, NE, Journal Star*, p 6; see also Bundesen, Herman (March 13, 1957). "Nervous Tension Eased by Tranquilizing Drugs." *Elizabethton, TN, Star*, p 4.

155 **NIMH psychiatrist Lawrence Kolb:** "Tranquilizer Drugs Are Held Harmful" (December 19, 1956). *New York Times*, p 33.

155 **others found that:** Abou-Setta, A. M., S. S. Mousavi, C. Spooner, et al. (August 2012). "First-Generation Versus Second-Generation Antipsychotics in Adults: Comparative Effectiveness." *Comparative Effectiveness Reviews* 63. Available here: https://www.ncbi.nlm.nih.gov/books/NBK107237/. Retrieved October 3, 2022.

156 **Still others would claim:** Chouinard, Guy, et al. (1978). "Neuroleptic-induced Supersensitivity Psychosis." *American Journal of Psychiatry* 135.11, p 1409. https://www.madinamerica.com/wp-content/uploads/2011/12/Chouinard%282%29pdf.pdf. Retrieved October 3, 2022; see also Muller, Pavel, and Philip Seeman (1978). "Dopaminergic Supersensitivity After Neuroleptics: Time-Course and Specificity." *Psychopharmacology*

60, pp 1–11. Available here: https://www.madinamerica.com/wp-content/uploads/2011/12/Muller.pdf. Retrieved October 3, 2022.

156 **Enthralled by the idea:** Horgan, John (1999). *The Undiscovered Mind: How the Human Brain Defies Replication, Medication, and Explanation.* New York: Touchstone, p 110.

156 **In the likes of Thorazine:** Caponi, Sandra (July 2021). "On the So-Called Psychopharmacological Revolution: The Discovery of Chlorpromazine and the Management of Madness." *História, Cie?ncias, Saúde* 28.3, p 2. Available here: https://www.scielo.br/j/hcsm/a/dWkfXqtyzGDsWMzPzCMcvZF/?format=pdf&lang=en. Retrieved October 3, 2022.

162 **President Kennedy had a plan:** Kennedy, John F. (May 25, 1961). "The Decision to Go to the Moon." National Aeronautics and Space Administration History Office. Available here: https://history.nasa.gov/moondec.html. Retrieved October 3, 2022.

162 **Kennedy signed into law:** Public Law 88-164. October 31, 1963. Available here: https://www.govinfo.gov/content/pkg/STATUTE-77/pdf/STATUTE-77-Pg282.pdf. Retrieved October 3, 2022.

162 **In a speech about:** Kennedy, John F. (October 31, 1963). "Remarks Upon Signing Bill for the Construction of Mental Retardation Facilities and Community Mental Health Centers." Online by Gerhard Peters and John T. Woolley, The American Presidency Project. https://www.presidency.ucsb.edu/documents/remarks-upon-signing-bill-for-the-construction-mental-retardation-facilities-and-community. Retrieved October 3, 2022.

162 **whose intellectual disability:** Shriver, Eunice Kennedy (1962). "Hope for Retarded Children." *Saturday Evening Post,* pp 71–75. Available here: http://www.saturdayeveningpost.com/wp-content/uploads/satevepost/1962-eunice-kennedy.pdf. Retrieved on October 3, 2022.

162 **To close the door:** Smith, Matthew (August 1, 2015). "An Ounce of Prevention." *Lancet* 386.9992, pp 424–25. Available here: https://www.thelancet.com/journals/lancet/article/PIIS0140-6736(15)61437-4/fulltext. Retrieved on October 3, 2022.

CHAPTER TWELVE

164 **King himself used the term:** Metzl, Jonathan (2010). *The Protest Psychosis: How Schizophrenia Became a Black Disease.* Boston: Beacon, p 121.

164 **But for psychiatrists:** Metzl 120–21.

164 **After spending twenty-four years:** Solomon, Jolie (March 21, 2022). "Overlooked No More: Louise Little, Activist and Mother of Malcolm X." *New York Times.* https://www.nytimes.com/2022/03/19/obituaries/louise-little-overlooked.html. Retrieved October 3, 2022.

165 **The state would later send:** Tubbs, Anna Malaika (2021). *The Three Mothers: How the Mothers of Martin Luther King, Jr., Malcolm X, and James Baldwin Shaped a Nation.* New York: Flatiron, p 189.

165 **pharmaceutical companies swiftly tapped:** Metzl 102–03.

166 **Rosenthal proposed that some inherited factor:** Rosenthal, David (1963). "Possible Environmental Factors: Prenatal Influences." In *The Genain Quadruplets: A Case Study and Theoretical Analysis of Heredity and Environment in Schizophrenia.* Ed. David Rosenthal. New York: Basic Books, p 574.

166 **"Nora," "Iris," "Myra," and "Hester":** Rosenthal, David (1963). "Introduction." In *The Genain Quadruplets: A Case Study and Theoretical Analysis of Heredity and Environment in Schizophrenia.* Ed. David Rosenthal. New York: Basic Books, p 9.

166 **he noted the "widespread psychiatric disorders":** Rosenthal, David (1963). "Possible Inherited Factors: EEG Abnormality." In *The Genain Quadruplets: A Case Study and Theoretical Analysis of Heredity and Environment in Schizophrenia.* Ed. David Rosenthal. New York: Basic Books, p 512.

166 **the quadruplets' own exhibition:** Rosenthal, David (1963). "The Nature of the Heredity-Environment Interaction." In *The Genain Quadruplets: A Case Study and Theoretical Analysis of Heredity and Environment in Schizophrenia.* Ed. David Rosenthal. New York: Basic Books, p 578.

166 **His chosen pseudonym:** Rosenthal, "Introduction," 9.

166 **"an unhappy collusion of nature and nurture":** Rosenthal, David (1963). "Possible Inherited Factors: Patterns of Behavioral Disturbance, Premorbid Personality, and Test Performance." In *The Genain Quadruplets: A Case Study and Theoretical Analysis of Heredity and Environment in Schizophrenia.* Ed. David Rosenthal. New York: Basic Books, p 534.

166 **Citing Paul Meehl's model:** Rosenthal, David (1963). "A Suggested Conceptual Framework." In *The Genain Quadruplets: A Case Study and Theoretical Analysis of Heredity and Environment in Schizophrenia.* Ed. David Rosenthal. New York: Basic Books, pp 507–08.

166 **Both parents "practiced" irrationality:** Rosenthal, David (1963). "Possible Environmental Factors: Life-Experience." In *The Genain Quadruplets: A Case Study and Theoretical Analysis of Heredity and Environment in Schizophrenia.* Ed. David Rosenthal. New York: Basic Books, p 560.

166 **there were both vertical and horizontal identification patterns:** Rosenthal, "Possible Environmental Factors: Life-Experience," 563.

166 **They tended to echo:** Rosenthal, "Possible Environmental Factors: Life-Experience," 564.

166 **Building on the work:** Rosenthal, "Possible Environmental Factors: Life-Experience," 551–52.

167 **Rosenthal also gestured toward:** Rosenthal, "Possible Environmental Factors: Life-Experience," 565.

167 **Bettelheim had argued:** Bettelheim, Bruno (1943). "Individual and Mass Behavior in Extreme Situations." *Journal of Abnormal and Social Psychology* 38.4, pp 417–52. https://pages.uoregon.edu/dluebke/HolocaustMemory407/Bettelheim1943.pdf.

167 **The quadruplets were "overpowered":** Rosenthal, "Possible Environmental Factors: Life-Experience," 548.

167 **Their mother surely smothered them:** Rosenthal, "Possible Environmental Factors: Life-Experience," 547.

167 **"provided no truly comforting respite":** Rosenthal, "Possible Environmental Factors: Life-Experience," 568.

167 **"remarkable balance":** Gottesman, Irving (January 9, 1965). "Theory of Schizophrenia." *British Medical Journal*, p 114. https://www.ncbi.nlm.nih.gov/pmc/articles/PMC2165039/pdf/brmedj02376-0070c.pdf.

168 **So did Leonard Heston:** Heston, Leonard L. (1966). "Psychiatric Disorders in Foster Home Reared Children of Schizophrenic Mothers." *British Journal of Psychiatry* 112, pp 819–25. Available here: https://www.gwern.net/docs/genetics/heritable/1966-heston.pdf.

168 **In 1966, Heston published:** Heston 825.

168 **Though he admitted:** Heston 821.

168 **though he never specified:** Heston 822.

168 **reached the threshold:** Joseph, Jay (March 2000). "Inaccuracy and Bias in Textbooks Reporting Psychiatric Research: The Case of the Schizophrenia Adoption Studies." *Politics and the Life Sciences* 19.1, p 92.

168 **Kety conceived of another approach:** Holzman, Philip S. (2001). "Seymour S. Kety and the Genetics of Schizophrenia." *Neuropsychopharmacology* 25.3, pp 299–300. Available here: https://www.nature.com/articles/1395719.pdf. Retrieved October 3, 2022.

168 **the government had constructed:** Harrington, Anne (2019). *Mind Fixers: Psychiatry's Troubled Search for the Biology of Mental Illness.* New York: Norton, p 172.

169 **NIMH's administrative control:** Low, Leanne (September–October 2021). "St. Elizabeths Hospital: How Its Architecture Informs Us of the Past and Present." *Catalyst* 29.5. https://irp.nih.gov/catalyst/v29i5/st-elizabeths-hospital. Retrieved October 3, 2022.

169 **delved deeper into:** Nagler, Shmuel, and Allan F. Mirsky (1985). "Introduction: The Israeli High-Risk Study." *Schizophrenia Bulletin* 11.1, pp 19–28. Available here: https://books.google.com/books?id=wlv0z9HCNzYC&pg=PA25&lpg=PA25&dq=david+rosenthal+kibbutz+studies+schizophrenia&source=bl&ots=V2OyU2IIKb&sig=ACfU3U2TBcRkZ3BHPAsCuwmprG3OjgBWuQ&hl=en&sa=X&ved=2ahUKEwjvzb-Ty-XzAhXegXIEHeA_AiQQ6AF6BAgOEAM#v=onepage&q=david%20rosenthal%20kibbutz%20studies%20schizophrenia&f=false. Retrieved October 3, 2022.

169 **Kety, Rosenthal, Wender, and a team:** Kety, S. S., D. Rosenthal, P. H. Wender, and F. Schulsinger (1968). "The Types and Prevalence of Mental Illness in the Biological and Adoptive Families of Adopted Schizophrenics." In *The Transmission of Schizophrenia*. Ed. D. Rosenthal and S. S. Kety. Oxford, UK: Pergamon Press, pp 347–49.

169 **There were thirty-three patients:** Kety, Rosenthal, Wender, and Schulsinger 349.

169 **The researchers then hunted:** Kety, Rosenthal, Wender, and Schulsinger 351.

169 **Much to the primary investigators' surprise:** Kety, Rosenthal, Wender, and Schulsinger 353–54; see also Harrington (2019) 173.

169 **Kety and his associates suggested:** Kety, Rosenthal, Wender, and Schulsinger 353.

170 **By broadening the diagnostic framework:** Kety, Rosenthal, Wender, and Schulsinger 353.

170 **More than half of the relatives:** Kety, Rosenthal, Wender, and Schulsinger 359.

170 **The researchers also utilized:** Rosenthal, D., P. H. Wender, S. S. Kety, F. Schulsinger, J. Welner, and L. Ostergaard (1968). "Schizophrenics' Offspring Reared in Adoptive Homes." In *The Transmission of Schizophrenia*. Ed. D. Rosenthal and S. S. Kety. Oxford, UK: Pergamon Press, p 377.

170 **Looking only at the subjects':** Rosenthal, Wender, Kety, Schulsinger, Welner, and Ostergaard 386–87.

170 **Kety and Rosenthal first introduced:** Harrington (2019) 173.

171 **Only the year before:** Parloff, Morris (2002 B). Interview by Ingrid Farreras. Office of NIH History and Stetten Museum. https://history.nih.gov/display/history/Parloff%2C+Morris+2002+B. Retrieved October 3, 2022; see also Zahn, Theodore Paul (December 19, 2001). Interview by Dr. Ingrid Farreras. Office of NIH History and Stetten Museum. https://history.nih.gov/display/history/Zahn%2C+Theodore+Paul+2001. Retrieved October 3, 2022.

171 **According to Carlos Sluzki:** Sluzki, Carlos (2007). "Lyman C. Wynne and the Transformation of the Field of Family-and-Schizophrenia." *Family Process* 46.2, pp 143–49. Available here: https://sluzki.com/publications/articles/147/lyman-c-wynne-and-the-transformation-of-the-field-of-family-and-schizophrenia. Retrieved October 3, 2022.

172 **If this elated:** Lidz, Theodore (1976). "Commentary on 'A Critical Review of Recent Adoption, Twin, and Family Studies of Schizophrenia.'" *Schizophrenia Bulletin* 2.3, pp 403–04.

172 **Lidz also criticized:** Lidz (1976) 407.

172 **Lidz was part of a small:** Shafti, Saeed Shoja (July 9, 2021). "Antipsychiatry Against Psychiatry: Remonstrations vs. Responsibilities." *Journal of Psychiatry Research* 3.3, p 3.

172 **While this view inclined Lidz:** Lidz (1976) 404.

172 **nor the notion:** Lidz, Theodore (Spring 1971). "Schizophrenia, R. D. Laing, and the Contemporary Treatment of Psychosis: An Interview with Dr. Theodore Lidz." Interviewed by Robert Orrill and Robert Boyers. *Salmagundi* 16, pp 19–130.

172 **He simply didn't think:** Lidz (1976) 404.

172 **Other so-called anti-psychiatrists:** Staub, Michael E. (2011). *Madness Is Civilization: When the Diagnosis Was Social, 1948–1980.* Chicago: University of Chicago Press, pp 59–60.

173 **The resistance to considering:** Metzl 96–97.

173 **Prior to leaving the institute:** McDaniel, Susan H. (2012). "Lyman Wynne." International Society for Psychological and Social Approaches to Psychosis. http://www.isps.org/index.php/isps-membership/isps-honorary-members/item/56-lyman-wynne. Retrieved October 3, 2022.

173 **After becoming chief:** Lenzer, Jeanne (August 21, 2004). "Loren Mosher." *British Medical Journal* 329.7463, p 463. https://www.ncbi.nlm.nih.gov/pmc/articles/PMC514223/. Retrieved October 3, 2022.

174 **NIMH formed the Center for Minority Group Mental Health Programs:** The Black Psychiatrists of America, "History." https://www.blackpsychiatrists.org/about. Retrieved October 3, 2022.

174 **the Black Psychiatrists of America:** https://www.blackpsychiatrists.org/about. Retrieved October 3, 2022.

174 **But even while officials declared:** Shapiro, Richard (Fall 1974). "Discrimination and Community Mental Health." *Civil Rights Digest*, p 22. Available here: https://books.google.com/books?id=AW5B1b_UJ-8C&pg=RA5-PA23&lpg=RA5-PA23&dq=#v=onepage&q&f=false. Retrieved October 3, 2022.

174 **was slow to diversify its ranks:** Carew, Jean (1977). "NIMH Policies Affecting Minorities." In *Minorities in Science: The Challenge for Change in Biomedicine*. Ed. Vijaya L. Melnick and Franklin D. Hamilton. New York: Plenum Press, p 110.

174 **staff members (including Kety) disparaged:** Kety, Seymour S. (1996). "Seymour S. Kety." In *The History of Neuroscience in Autobiography*, volume 1. Ed. Larry R. Squire. Washington, DC: Society for Neuroscience, p 406.

174 **both internal scientists and external grants:** Whitaker, Robert (2010). *Anatomy of an Epidemic: Magic Bullets, Psychiatric Drugs, and the Astonishing Rise of Mental Illness in America.* New York: Crown, p 272; see also Zahn.

174 **looking, for instance, at the outcomes:** Whitaker (2010) 96.

174 **Researchers routinely championed:** Whitaker, Robert (2001). *Mad in America: Bad Science, Bad Medicine, and the Enduring Mistreatment of the Mentally Ill.* New York: Basic Books, pp 157–58, 181–82.

174 **NIMH researchers also discouraged:** Whitaker (2001) 158.

174 **So claimed a researcher in 1967:** Seeman, Mary V. (July 19, 2021). "History of the Dopamine Hypothesis of Antipsychotic Action." *World Journal of Psychiatry* 11.7, pp 355–64.

174 **According to medical journalist:** Whitaker (2010) 78.

175 **Black Americans were more likely:** Metzl, Jonathan (January 25, 2010). "In Medical Records, a Story of the Racialization of Schizophrenia." *Beacon Broadside.* https://www.beaconbroadside.com/broadside/2010/01/jonathan-metzl-in-medical-records-a-story-of-the-racialization-of-schizophrenia.html. Retrieved on October 3, 2022.

175 **By 1975, the population:** Lindamood, Wes (June 20, 2005). "Thorazine. Purpose Antipsychotic." *Chemical and Engineering News* 83.25. https://cen.acs.org/articles/83/i25/Thorazine.html. Retrieved on October 3, 2022.

175 **Many who needed intensive treatment:** Torrey, E. Fuller (2013). *American Psychosis: How the Federal Government Destroyed the Mental Illness Treatment System.* Oxford, UK, and New York: Oxford University Press, pp 78–79.

175 **Presenting forced hospitalization:** Torrey (2013) 71–72, 86.

175 **President Lyndon B. Johnson secured the passage:** Scull, Andrew (Winter 2021). "'Community Care': Historical Perspective on Deinstitutionalization." *Perspectives in Biology and Medicine* 64.1, p 74.

176 **These programs did not pay benefits:** Scull 75.

176 **In California:** Torrey, E. Fuller (September 9, 2013). "Ronald Reagan's Shameful Legacy: Violence, the Homeless, Mental Illness." *Salon.* https://www.salon.com/2013/09/29/ronald_reagans_shameful_legacy_violence_the_homeless_mental_illness/. Retrieved October 3, 2022.

176 **When Social Security Disability Insurance (SSDI) became available:** Scull 75–76.

176 **Sociologist Andrew Scull observed:** Quoted in Torrey (2013).

176 **An average day for a patient:** Scull 76.

177 **ceased taking their medications:** Torrey, E. Fuller, and Mary T. Zdanowicz (July 9, 1999). "Deinstitutionalization Hasn't Worked." *Washington Post.* https://www.washingtonpost.com/archive/opinions/1999/07/09/deinstitutionalization-hasnt-worked/31574935-984f-41a6-ba0b-55b071cf8b4c/. Retrieved October 3, 2022.

178 **according to a letter:** Rosenthal, David (May 10, 1965). Letter to Dave Shakow. From Scott Rosenthal's collection.

179 **The institutional reform began:** Parloff (2002 B).

179 **This decision came after:** National Institute of Mental Health (October 21, 2021). *NIH Almanac.* https://www.nih.gov/about-nih/what-we-do/nih-almanac/national-institute-mental-health-nimh. Retrieved October 3, 2022.

179 **These realignments reflected:** Ingraham, Loring (December 9, 2002). Interview by Ingrid Farreras. Office of NIH History and Stetten Museum. https://history.nih.gov/display/history/Ingraham%2C+Loring+2002. Retrieved October 3, 2022.

179 **Perceiving this new directive:** Zahn.

180 **Not even Parloff suspected:** Parloff (2002 B).

180 **By the late '70s:** Ingraham.

180 **a colleague named Virgil Carlson reached out:** Carlson, Virgil (March 21, 2002). Interview by Ingrid Farreras. Office of NIH History and Stetten Museum. https://history.nih.gov/display/history/Carlson%2C+Virgil+2002. Retrieved October 3, 2022.

CHAPTER THIRTEEN

186 **As Rosenthal put it:** Rosenthal, David (1963). "Possible Environmental Factors: Life-Experience." In *The Genain Quadruplets: A Case Study and Theoretical Analysis of Heredity and Environment in Schizophrenia*. Ed. David Rosenthal. New York: Basic Books, p 559.

187 **Anthropologist Jules Henry:** Staub, Michael E. (2011). *Madness Is Civilization: When the Diagnosis Was Social, 1948–1980.* Chicago: University of Chicago Press, p 59.

187 **"It is clear":** Staub 60.

187 **Such a theory attempted:** Staub 59.

187 **Malcom X had declared:** Metzl, Jonathan (2014). "Controllin the Planet."

Transition 115, p 30. Available here: https://www.vanderbilt.edu/mhs/wp-content/uploads/sites/181/transition.115.231.pdf. Retrieved on October 3, 2022.

187 **the social critic and literary icon James Baldwin:** Baldwin, James (October 16, 1963). "A Talk to Teachers." Delivered October 16, 1963, as "The Negro Child—His Self-Image." Originally published in *The Saturday Review* (December 21, 1963). https://www.spps.org/cms/lib010/MN01910242/Centricity/Domain/125/baldwin_atalktoteachers_1_2.pdf. Retrieved on October 3, 2022.

188 **R. D. Laing elaborated upon:** Laing, R. D. (1967). *The Politics of Experience and The Bird of Paradise.* New York: Penguin, p 113.

188 **The function of the family:** Laing 65.

188 **Laing revived the work:** Laing, R. D. (1993). "Why Is Reich Never Mentioned?" *Pulse of the Planet* 4, pp 76–77. Available here: http://www.orgonelab.org/LaingOnReich.pdf. Retrieved on October 3, 2022.

188 **For Reich, Germans had chosen:** Schatzman, Morton (1973). *Soul Murder: Persecution in the Family.* New York: Random House, p 75. Based on Reich, William (1946). *The Mass Psychology of Fascism.* Trans. Theodore P. Wolfe. New York: Orgone Institute Press. Available here: https://ia801603.us.archive.org/25/items/WilhelmReichTheMassPsychologyOfFascism_20170308/Wilhelm%20Reich%20-%20The%20Mass%20Psychology%20of%20Fascism.pdf. Retrieved on October 3, 2022.

189 **American feminists were also:** Brownmiller, Susan (January 26, 2009). "The Woman Who Fought Freud—and Won." Women's Media Center. https://womensmediacenter.com/news-features/the-woman-who-fought-freudand-won. Retrieved on October 3, 2022.

189 **For these bold claims:** Beck, Richard (2015). *We Believe the Children: A Moral Panic in the 1980s.* New York: Public Affairs, p 7.

189 **The National Organization of Women then took up her call:** Beck 8.

189 **He subsequently signed:** Beck 9.

189 **In 1975, a new edition:** Beck 24.

189 **stated that familial incest:** Kluft, Richard P. (January 12, 2011). "Ramifications of Incest." *Psychiatric Times* 27.12. https://www.psychiatrictimes.com/view/ramifications-incest. Retrieved on October 3, 2022.

189 **But Rush refused:** Beck 15–16.

190 **For all her indignation:** Bromberg, Eli (2020). *Unsettling: Jews, Whiteness, and Incest in American Popular Culture.* New Brunswick, NJ: Rutgers University Press, p 14.

190 **With the exception of Betty Friedan's:** Bromberg 19.

190 **disappear into whiteness:** Bromberg 34.

190 **While these contributors frowned:** Rosenthal, "Possible Environmental Factors: Life-Experience," 568.

191 **Perturbed that psychiatry had succeeded:** Szasz, Thomas (1960). "The Myth of Mental Illness." *American Psychologist* 15, pp 113–18. Available here: https://depts.washington.edu/psychres/wordpress/wp-content/uploads/2017/07/100-Papers-in-Clinical-Psychiatry-Conceptual-issues-in-psychiatry-The-Myth-of-Mental-Illness.pdf. Retrieved on October 3, 2022.

191 **British social theorist Peter Sedgwick made:** Sedgwick, Peter (1982). *Psycho-Politics.* London: Pluto, p 175.

191 **For critics like Sedgwick:** See part 2 of Sedgwick for a critique of libertarian anti-psychiatry. Cf. "The libertarian posture in mental health shields those who adopt it from demanding and assuming the responsibility for a continuing care for the disabled," p 248.

192 **the Gipper slashed federal benefits:** Staub 184.

192 **On the campaign trail:** Levin, Josh (December 19, 2013). "The Welfare Queen." *Slate.* http://www.slate.com/articles/news_and_politics/history/2013/12/linda_taylor_welfare_queen_ronald_reagan_made_her_a_notorious_american_villain.html. Retrieved on October 3, 2022.

192 **broader GOP strategy:** Perlstein, Rick (November 13, 2012). "Exclusive: Lee Atwater's Infamous 1981 Interview on the Southern Strategy." *The Nation.* https://www.thenation.com/article/archive/exclusive-lee-atwaters-infamous-1981-interview-southern-strategy/. Retrieved on October 3, 2022. Note: Atwater denies Reagan used dog whistles, but scholars view Reagan as having perfected the rhetorical technique that Atwater attributes to Nixon and others. See, for example, Haney-Lopez, Ian (January 1, 2011). "The Racism at the Heart of the Reagan Presidency." *Salon.* https://www.salon.com/2014/01/11/the_racism_at_the_heart_of_the_reagan_presidency/. Retrieved on October 3, 2022.

192 **Following the cancellation:** Staub 184.

192 **Making matters worse:** Torrey, E. Fuller (September 9, 2013). "Ronald Reagan's Shameful Legacy: Violence, the Homeless, Mental Illness." *Salon.* https://www.salon.com/2013/09/29/ronald_reagans_shameful_legacy_violence_the_homeless_mental_illness/. Retrieved October 3, 2022.

192 **The dollars were diverted:** Anderson, James R. (1981). "Bankrupting America: The Impact of President Reagan's Military Budget." *International Journal of Health Services* 11.4, pp 623–29.

192 **soon-to-be-privatized jails:** Abood, Mitchell (January 31, 2021). "The Evolution of Private Prison Incarceration in the United States." *University of Miami Law Review* 75. https://lawreview.law.miami.edu/evolution-private-prison-incarceration-united-states/. Retrieved on October 3, 2022.

192 **In the wake of the funding cuts:** Staub 184.

193 **One of these was:** Torrey (2013).

193 **As news coverage:** Staub 185.

193 **"I think some people are going":** McFadden, Robert D. (December 10, 1983). "Comments by Meese on Hunger Produce a Storm of Controversy." *New York Times*, p 12.

193 **The president echoed:** Jones, Marian Moser (March 2015). "Creating a Science of Homelessness During the Reagan Era." *Milbank Quarterly* 93.1, pp 139–78.

193 **Reaganism further transformed:** Holden, Constance. "Reagan Versus the Social Sciences." *Science* 226.4678, pp 1052–54; see also Miller, Roberta Balstad (2002). "Crisis and Responses: The Politics of the Social Sciences in the United States (1980–

1982)." *La biologie* 7; and Zahn, Theodore Paul (December 19, 2001). Interview by Dr. Ingrid Farreras. Office of NIH History and Stetten Museum. https://history.nih.gov/display/history/Zahn%2C+Theodore+Paul+2001. Retrieved October 3, 2022.

195 **Rosenthal's successor and his crew:** DeLisi, Lynn E., et al. (1984). "The Genain Quadruplets 25 Years Later: A Diagnostic and Biochemical Followup." *Psychiatry Research* 31.1, p 59.

195 **published the first of a three-paper series:** DeLisi 59.

195 **Off medication, the women did:** DeLisi 71–73.

196 **In the second paper:** Mirsky, Allan F. (2019). "Monte S. Buchsbaum and the Genain Quadruplets." *Psychiatry Research* 277, pp 70–71.

197 **Mirsky et al. published a third:** Mirsky, Allan F., et al. (1984). "The Genain Quadruplets: Psychological Studies." *Psychiatry Research* 13.1, pp 77–93.

197 **Four years later:** Mirsky, Allan F., and Olive W. Quinn (1988). "The Genain Quadruplets." *Schizophrenia Bulletin* 14.4, p 595.

197 **By this, they primarily meant:** Mirsky and Quinn 607–08.

CHAPTER FOURTEEN

200 **"I always thought":** Cohen, Robert A. (2002 C). Interview by Ingrid Farreras. Office of NIH History and Stetten Museum. https://history.nih.gov/display/history/Cohen%2C+Robert+A.+2002+C. Retrieved on October 3, 2022.

200 **According to Cohen:** Cohen, Robert A. (January 18, 2002 A). Interview by Ingrid Farreras. Office of NIH History and Stetten Museum. https://history.nih.gov/display/history/Cohen%2C+Robert+A.+2002+A. Retrieved on October 3, 2022.

200 **And following Allan Mirsky's appointment:** Coppola, Richard (December 11, 2002). Interview by Ingrid Farreras. Office of NIH History and Stetten Museum. https://history.nih.gov/display/history/Coppola%2C+Richard+2002. Retrieved on October 3, 2022.

201 **Evolutionary geneticist Richard Lewontin:** Lewontin, Richard, Steven Rose, and Leon Kamin (1984). *Not in Our Genes: Biology, Ideology and Human Nature.* New York: Pantheon, p xv.

201 **closely examined:** Lewontin, Rose, and Kamin 222–23.

202 **As Lewontin, Rose, and Kamin explained:** Lewontin, Rose, and Kamin 223.

203 **Combing through data:** Lewontin, Rose, and Kamin 224.

203 **Lewontin, Rose, and Kamin could "only marvel":** Lewontin, Rose, and Kamin 225.

203 **Kenneth S. Kendler and Alan M. Gruenberg released:** Kendler, Kenneth S., and Alan M. Gruenberg (June 1984). "An Independent Analysis of the Danish Adoption Study of Schizophrenia." *Archives of General Psychiatry* 41, p 556.

204 **who actually found:** Kendler and Gruenberg 564.

204 **Seven years later:** Breggin, Peter (1991). *Toxic Psychiatry: Why Therapy, Empathy and Love Must Replace the Drugs, Electroshock, and Biochemical Theories of the "New Psychiatry."* New York: St. Martin's, p 98.

205 **The Center for Minority Group Mental Health Programs:** Brown, Bertram S., and K. Patrick Okura (2015). *Mental Health, Racism, and Sexism.* Ed. Charles V. Willi, Patricia Perri Rieker, Bernard M. Kramer, and Bertram S. Brown. Pittsburgh: University of Pittsburgh Press, pp 415–16.

205 **NIMH dismissed Mosher:** Bernstein, Adam (July 20, 2004). "Contrarian Psychiatrist Loren Mosher, 70." *Washington Post*, p B06. Available here: https://www.washingtonpost.com/wp-dyn/articles/A63107-2004Jul19.html. Retrieved October 3, 2022.

205 **In the wake of:** "Physical Security Project Requirements for NIH Owned and Leased Facilities." NIH Policy Manual. https://policymanual.nih.gov/1381. Retrieved October 3, 2022.

CHAPTER FIFTEEN

210 **evangelical Christian psychologist James Dobson:** Du Mez, Kristin Kobes (2020). *Jesus and John Wayne: How White Evangelicals Corrupted a Faith and Fractured a Nation.* New York: Norton, 79–80.

210 **while he was still working:** Farley, Audrey Clare (May 12, 2021). "The Eugenics Roots of Evangelical Family Values." *Religion & Politics.* https://religionandpolitics.org/2021/05/12/the-eugenics-roots-of-evangelical-family-values/. Retrieved on October 3, 2022; see also Stephens, Hilde Løvdal (2019). *Family Matters: James Dobson and Focus on the Family's Crusade for the Christian Home.* Tuscaloosa: University of Alabama Press.

210 **"a marvelous purifier":** Dobson, James (1970). *Dare to Discipline.* Wheaton, IL: Tyndale House, p 27.

210 **"a little bit of pain [went] a long way":** Dobson (1970) 35.

210 **with "sufficient magnitude":** Dobson (1970) 35.

210 **Here he described:** Dobson, James (1978). *The Strong Willed Child: Birth Through Adolescence.* Wheaton, IL: Tyndale House, pp 1–9.

211 **also recommended squeezing:** Dobson (1978) 138.

211 **leaving paddles:** Dobson (1978) 62.

211 **By quoting these passages:** Dobson (1978) 7, 61, 235.

211 **taking great care:** Dobson (1978) 28.

211 **According to journalist Talia Lavin:** Lavin, Talia (November 8, 2021). "Corporal Punishment, Evangelicals, and the Doctrine of Obedience." *The Sword & the Sandwich.* https://theswordandthesandwich.substack.com/p/ministry-of-violence-parts-iiii. Retrieved on October 3, 2022.

211 **Some also describe:** Lavin, Talia (November 1, 2021). "Love, Pain, and Evangelical Corporal Punishment." *The Sword and the Sandwich.* https://theswordandthesandwich.substack.com/p/ministry-of-violence-part-ii. Retrieved on October 3, 2022.

211 **Gothard and his colleagues toured:** "History." Institute in Basic Life Principles. https://iblp.org/about-iblp/iblp-history. Retrieved on October 3, 2022.

212 **Building on the "dominionist" philosophy:** Du Mez 75–76.

212 **Gothard did not desire:** Images of Gothard's "wisdom booklets," suggesting democracy is ineffective and unbiblical, recently went viral. Stern, Carly (February 19, 2021). "Ex-Evangelical Reveals She Was Taught That Democracy Is 'Fundamentally Bad'." *Daily Mail.* https://www.dailymail.co.uk/femail/article-9278709/Ex-evangelical-reveals-homeschool-materials-given-child-say-democracy-bad.html. Retrieved on October 3, 2022.

212 **Farris, for his part, advised:** Huseman, Jessica (August 27, 2015). "The Frightening Power of the Home-Schooling Lobby." *Slate.* https://slate.com/human-interest/2015/08/home-school-legal-defense-association-how-a-home-schooling-group-fights-any-meaningful-regulations-of-families-that-pull-their-kids-from-school.html. Retrieved on October 3, 2022; and Stollar, R. L. (2014). "Children as Divine Rental Property: An Exposition of HSLDA's Philosophy of Parental Rights." Homeschool Alumni Reaching Out. Available here: https://homeschoolersanonymous.files.wordpress.com/2015/01/childrenasproperty.pdf. Retrieved on October 3, 2022.

212 **later going so far:** Farris, Michael (2001). *Forbid Them Not.* Nashville: B&H Publishing.

213 **The hullabaloo began:** Smith, Michelle, and Lawrence Pazder (1980). *Michelle Remembers.* New York: St. Martin's; see also Goodwin, Megan (2018). "They Couldn't Get My Soul: Recovered Memories, Ritual Abuse, and the Specter(s) of Religious Difference." *Studies in Religion* 247.2, p 283.

213 **Smith's father claimed:** Grescoe, Paul (October 27, 1980). "Things That Go Bump in Victoria." *Maclean's.* https://archive.macleans.ca/article/1980/10/27/things-that-go-bump-in-victoria. Retrieved on October 3, 2022.

213 **There was, for instance:** Beck, Richard (2015). *We Believe the Children: A Moral Panic in the 1980s.* New York: Public Affairs, p 26.

213 **A school yearbook showed:** Beck 27.

213 **Catapulted to international fame:** Goodwin (2018) 287.

214 **a mother claimed:** McPadden, Mike (July 25, 2019). "What You Need to Know About the Bizarre McMartin Preschool Satanic Sex Abuse Trials." *Investigation Discovery Crime-Feed* (blog). https://www.investigationdiscovery.com/crimefeed/crime-history/5-facts-you-need-to-know-about-the-mcmartin-preschool-satanic-sex-abuse-trial. Retrieved on October 3, 2022; see also Yuhas, Alan (March 31, 2021). "It's Time to Revisit the Satanic Panic." *New York Times.* https://www.nytimes.com/2021/03/31/us/satanic-panic.html. Retrieved on October 3, 2022.

214 **parents then interrogated:** Beck 36.

214 **The police hired therapists:** Yuhas.

214 **children began to tell:** Goodwin, Megan (2020). *Abusing Religion: Literary Persecution, Sex Scandals, and Minority Religions.* New Brunswick, NJ: Rutgers University Press, p 35.

214 **orgies, child sacrifice:** McPadden.

214 **a former lobbyist:** van Til, Reinder (1997). *Lost Daughters: Recovered Memory Therapy and the People It Hurts.* Grand Rapids, MI: Eerdman's, p 134.

214 **used anatomically correct dolls:** Beck 41.

214 **praising those who reported misdeeds:** Coleman, Lee (Spring 1989). "Learning from the McMartin Hoax." *Institute for Psychological Therapies Journal* 1.2. Available here: http://www.ipt-forensics.com/journal/volume1/j1_2_7.htm. Retrieved on October 3, 2022.

214 **She then went before Congress:** MacFarlane, Kee (September 17, 1984). Joint Hearing Before the Subcommittee on Oversight of the Committee on Ways and Means and Select Committee on Children, Youth, and Families. House of Representatives. Ninety-Eighth Congress, Second Session. Available here: https://www.ojp.gov/pdffiles1/Digitization/107803NCJRS.pdf. Retrieved on October 3, 2022.

214 **Congress increased funding:** Nathan, Debbie, and Michael Snedeker (1995). *Satan's Silence: Ritual Abuse and the Making of a Modern American Witch Hunt.* San Jose, CA: Author's Choice, p 127.

214 **much of the money going:** Nathan and Snedeker 126.

215 **Congress also passed:** "Child Protection Act of 1984." https://www.congress.gov/bill/98th-congress/house-bill/3635. Retrieved on October 3, 2022.

215 **legislators weren't so interested:** Beck 8, 132, 138.

215 **it primarily emboldened:** Goodwin (2020) 58.

215 **it supplemented such efforts:** Eugenios, Jillian (April 13, 2022). "How 1970s Christian Crusader Anita Bryant Helped Spawn Florida's LGBTQ Culture War." *NBC News.* https://www.nbcnews.com/nbc-out/out-news/1970s-christian-crusader-anita-bryant-helped-spawn-floridas-lgbtq-cult-rcna24215. Retrieved on October 3, 2022.

215 **more than a hundred other:** Hughes, Sarah (August 2017). "American Monsters: Tabloid Media and the Satanic Panic, 1970–2000." *Journal of American Studies* 51.3, pp 691–719.

215 **individuals collectively lodged:** Goleman, Daniel (October 31, 1994). "Proof Lacking for Ritual Abuse by Satanists." https://web.archive.org/web/20180521193259/https://www.nytimes.com/1994/10/31/us/proof-lacking-for-ritual-abuse-by-satanists.html?sq=satanic+ritual+abuse&scp=1&st=nyt. Retrieved on October 3, 2022.

215 **Satanists were using:** Waldron, David (Spring 2005). "Role-Playing Games and the Christian Right: Community Formation in Response to a Moral Panic." *Journal of Religion and Popular Culture* 9. https://web.archive.org/web/20130104131941/http://www.usask.ca/relst/jrpc/art9-roleplaying-print.html. Retrieved on October 3, 2022.

215 **A network of Christian:** Goodwin (2018) 283, 286, 288.

216 **appealed to Christian professionals:** Beck 130.

216 **Secular professional societies were not:** Noll, Richard. "Speak, Memory." *Psychiatric Times.* https://www.psychiatrictimes.com/view/speak-memory. Retrieved on October 3, 2022.

216 **After MPD debuted:** Beck 126.

216 **into a childlike state of mind:** Goodwin (2018) 288.

217 **traditionalists were using:** Hughes, Sarah (2021). "The Perils of Punky: Gender,

Childhood, and the Occult." *American Tabloid Media and the Satanic Panic, 1970–2000.* New York: Palgrave, pp 159–213.

217 **many women's rights advocates:** Jarrett, Kelly Jo (2000). *Strange Bedfellows: Religion, Feminism, and Fundamentalism in the Satanic Panic.* PhD Dissertation, Duke University. Duke University ProQuest Dissertations Publishing. Available here: https://www.proquest.com/openview/d25a19974366d2617deeebf75f532479/1. Retrieved on October 3, 2022.

217 **Feminist icon:** Beck 211.

217 **prosecutors charged Buckey and six other McMartin employees:** McPadden.

217 **Journalist Geraldo Rivera aired:** Shales, Tom (October 27, 1988). "The Devil to Pay." *Washington Post.* https://www.washingtonpost.com/archive/lifestyle/1988/10/27/the-devil-to-pay/9b39d002-c2ae-42b7-82ae-e4794598142f/. Retrieved on October 3, 2022.

217 **screened before church congregations:** Victor, Jeffrey S. (1993). *Satanic Panic: The Creation of a Contemporary Legend.* Chicago: Open Court, p 46.

217 **he alleged that at least one million:** Lewis, James R. (2001). *Satanism Today: An Encyclopedia of Religion, Folklore, and Modern Culture.* Santa Barbara, CA: ABC-Clio, p 224.

217 **Smith and Pazder also lent a hand:** Goodwin (2020) 83.

217 **Still, there was not a single:** Timnick, Lois, and Carol McGraw (January 19, 1990). "McMartin Verdict: Not Guilty." *Los Angeles Times.* https://www.latimes.com/archives/la-xpm-1990-01-19-mn-223-story.html. Retrieved on October 3, 2022.

217 **Nor were there any:** Goleman.

218 **Though no one was convicted:** Goodwin (2018) 282.

218 **Some believers became so persuaded:** Young-Bruehl, Elisabeth (2012). *Childism: Confronting Prejudice Against Children.* New Haven, CT: Yale University Press, p 327.

218 **therapists would be exposed:** French, Christopher (July 13, 2015). "The Legacy of Implanted Satanic Abuse 'Memories' Is Still Causing Damage Today." *The Conversation.* https://theconversation.com/the-legacy-of-implanted-satanic-abuse-memories-is-still-causing-damage-today-43755. Retrieved on October 3, 2022.

218 **But the primary effects:** Goodwin (2018) abstract.

218 **None other than Gothard:** Bailey, Sarah Pulliam (January 6, 2016). "New Charges Allege Religious Leader, Who Has Ties to the Duggars, Sexually Abused Women." *Washington Post.* https://www.washingtonpost.com/news/acts-of-faith/wp/2016/01/06/new-charges-allege-religious-leader-who-has-ties-to-the-duggars-sexually-abused-women/. Retrieved on October 3, 2022.

218 **The Basic Youth Conflicts founder resigned:** Bailey.

218 **found no criminal activity:** Radnofsky, Caroline (February 6, 2022). "Ministry That Once Nourished Duggar Family's Faith Falls from Grace." *NBC News.* https://www.nbcnews.com/news/us-news/ministry-nourished-duggar-familys-faith-falls-grace-rcna14024. Retrieved on October 3, 2022.

218 **Farris defended Gothard:** Huseman, Nick Ducote (February 18, 2014). "Dear Michael Farris, Sexual Abuse Isn't a 'Basic Strength' That 'Can Get Out of Control.'" *Homeschool-*

ers Anonymous. https://homeschoolersanonymous.wordpress.com/2014/02/18/dear-michael-farris-sexual-abuse-isnt-a-basic-strength-that-can-get-out-of-control/. Retrieved on October 3, 2022.

218 **undercut legal safeguards:** Anne, Libby (April 17, 2013). "HSLDA's Fight against Child Abuse Reporting." *Patheos.* https://www.patheos.com/blogs/lovejoyfeminism/2013/04/hsldas-fight-against-child-abuse-reporting.html. Retrieved on October 3, 2022.

220 **a phenomenon well captured:** Sehgal, Parul (May 3, 2016). "The Forced Heroism of the 'Survivor.'" *New York Times.* https://www.nytimes.com/2016/05/08/magazine/the-forced-heroism-of-the-survivor.html. Retrieved on October 3, 2022.

220 **Sándor Ferenczi's concept:** Rachman, Arnold W. (December 1999). "Ferenczi's Rise and Fall from 'Analytic Grace': The Ferenczi Renaissance Revisited." *Group* 23.3/4, pp 108–09.

220 **The 1980s also saw the publication:** Sandomir, Richard (February 4, 2020). "Dr. Leonard Shengold, 94, Psychoanalyst Who Studied Child Abuse, Dies." *New York Times.* https://www.nytimes.com/2020/02/04/health/leonard-shengold-dead.html. Retrieved on October 3, 2022.

220 **which argued that "the righteousness and religiosity":** Shengold, Leonard (1991). *Soul Murder: The Effects of Childhood Abuse and Deprivation.* New York: Fawcett, Columbine, p 22.

220 **"compulsion to repeat":** Shengold 4–5.

220 **When parents presented:** Shengold 22.

220 **Curiously, Shengold also identified:** See Shengold chapters 5–7 on "rat people."

221 **which she deemed:** Miller, Alice (June 14, 2007). "Spanking as Sexual Abuse." https://www.alice-miller.com/en/spanking-as-sexual-abuse/. Retrieved on October 3, 2022.

221 **increased the risk of antisocial behaviors:** Miller, Alice (2015). "Spanking Is Counterproductive and Dangerous." https://www.alice-miller.com/en/spanking-is-counterproductive-and-dangerous/. Retrieved on October 3, 2022.

221 **Being spanked instilled the desire:** Miller, Alice (October 22, 1998). "The Childhood Trauma." http://www.vachss.com/guest_dispatches/alice_miller2.html. Retrieved on October 3, 2022.

221 **In the 1980s:** "Northville Psychiatric Hospital." Detroit Urbex. http://www.detroiturbex.com/content/healthandsafety/northville/index.html. Retrieved on October 3, 2022; see also the coverage of *Detroit Free Press*: Castine, John (December 18, 1982). "US to Check How Patients Are Treated at Northville." *Detroit Free Press*, p 3; and Kresnak, Jack (August 2, 1986). "Probe Investigates Possible Negligence in Northville Death." *Detroit Free Press*, p 3.

221 **With the flourishing of trauma studies:** Hartney, Elizabeth (February 16, 2022). "9 Reasons the Cycle of Abuse Continues." *Very Well Mind.* https://www.verywellmind.com/the-cycle-of-sexual-abuse-22460. Retrieved on October 3, 2022.

222 **Even in the majority of cases:** Atlas, Galit (2022). *Emotional Inheritance: A Therapist, Her Patients, and the Legacy of Trauma.* New York: Little, Brown.

223 **The federal government had initially:** Thomas, Karen Kruse (April 21, 2020).

“The Other Time a US President Withheld WHO Funds.” Bloomberg School of Public Health. https://publichealth.jhu.edu/2020/the-other-time-a-us-president-withheld-who-funds. Retrieved on October 3, 2022.

223 **President Reagan going four years:** Bennington-Castro, Joseph (June 1, 2020). “How AIDS Remained an Unspoken—But Deadly—Epidemic for Years.” History.com. https://www.history.com/news/aids-epidemic-ronald-reagan. Retrieved on October 3, 2022.

223 **Activists and the media forced:** Keeler, Maggie (December 1, 2021). “Remembering Ryan White’s Legacy on World AIDS Day.” *DC Health Matters* (blog). https://dchealthmattersblog.org/remembering-ryan-whites-legacy-on-world-aids-day/. Retrieved on October 3, 2022.

224 **Psychotherapist Galit Atlas:** Atlas 56–57.

225 **the concept appeared:** Phillips, Adam (1994). “Freud and the Uses of Forgetting.” In *On Flirtation*. Cambridge, MA: Harvard University Press, pp 33–35.

225 **when the government researchers formally studied:** Mirsky, Allan F., et al. (2000). “A 39-Year Followup of the Genain Quadruplets.” *Schizophrenia Bulletin* 26.3, pp 699–708.

226 **In a 2000 paper:** Mirsky et al. (2000) 699.

226 **For all his emphasis on biology:** Mirsky et al. (2000) 706.

226 **After reviewing the study:** “Four Sisters with Schizophrenia, Four Decades of Scrutiny” (October 2000). WebMD. https://www.webmd.com/schizophrenia/news/20001020/four-sisters-with-schizophrenia-four-decades-of-scrutiny. Retrieved on October 3, 2022.

227 **Mirsky noted:** Mirsky et al. (2000) 701.

227 **told *Science* magazine:** Hamer, Blythe (August 14, 1982). “Identical Quadruplet Sisters, All Schizophrenics, Prove Fascinating Source of Study.” *Kingston Whig-Standard*, p 23.

CHAPTER SIXTEEN

228 **Human Genome Project:** “Fact Sheet” (August 24, 2022). Human Genome Project Research Institute. https://www.genome.gov/human-genome-project/What. Retrieved on October 3, 2022.

228 **Estimated to take fifteen years:** “Completion FAQ.” Human Genome Project Research Institute. https://www.genome.gov/human-genome-project/Completion-FAQ. Retrieved on October 3, 2022.

228 **Early in the project:** St. Clair, David (May 30, 2021). “Schizophrenia: A Classic Battle Ground of Nature Versus Nurture Debate.” *Science Bulletin* 66.10, pp 1037–46.

229 **the findings were underwhelming:** Johnson, Emma C., et al. (November 15, 2017). “No Evidence That Schizophrenia Candidate Genes Are More Associated with Schizophrenia Than Non-Candidate Genes.” *Biological Psychiatry* 82.10, pp 702–08.

229 **Next came the genome-wide association studies:** St. Clair.

229 **GWAS have identified:** "Biological Insights from 108 Schizophrenia-Associated Genetic Loci" (2014). *Nature* 511, pp 421–27. https://www.nature.com/articles/nature13595. Retrieved on October 3, 2022; see also Henriksen, Mads G., Julie Nordgaard, and Lennart B. Jansson (June 22, 2017). "Genetics of Schizophrenia: Overview of Methods, Findings and Limitations." *Frontiers in Human Neuroscience.* Available here: https://www.frontiersin.org/articles/10.3389/fnhum.2017.00322/full. Retrieved on October 3, 2022.

229 **Because none of these:** Marsman, Anne, et al. (November 2020). "Do Current Measures of Polygenic Risk for Mental Disorders Contribute to Population Variance in Mental Health?" *Schizophrenia Bulletin* 46.6, pp 1353–62.

229 **polygenic score cards only explain:** Marsman.

229 **Though it is believed:** Fullerton, Janice M., et al. (2019). "Polygenic Risk Scores in Psychiatry: Will They Be Useful for Clinicians?" *F1000 Faculty Reviews* 8. Available here: https://www.ncbi.nlm.nih.gov/pmc/articles/PMC6676506/. Retrieved on October 3, 2022.

230 **Epigenetic mechanisms include:** Lacal, Irene, and Rossella Ventura (September 28, 2018). "Epigenetic Inheritance: Concepts, Mechanisms and Perspectives." *Frontiers in Molecular Neuroscience* 11, p 292. https://www.frontiersin.org/articles/10.3389/fnmol.2018.00292/full.

230 **A direct epigenetic mechanism believed:** Roth, Tania L., et al. (September 2009). "Epigenetic Mechanisms in Schizophrenia." *Biochemica et Biophysica* 1790.9, pp 869–77.

230 **researchers claimed:** Yehuda, Rachel, et al. (August 12, 2015). "Holocaust Exposure Induced Intergenerational Effects on FKBP5 Methylation." *Biological Psychiatry.* https://www.biologicalpsychiatryjournal.com/article/S0006-3223(15)00652-6/fulltext. Retrieved on October 3, 2022.

230 **But some believe the investigators:** Yasmin, Seema (June 9, 2017). "Experts Debunk Study That Found Holocaust Trauma Is Inherited." *Chicago Tribune.* https://www.chicagotribune.com/lifestyles/health/ct-holocaust-trauma-not-inherited-20170609-story.html. Retrieved on October 3, 2022.

230 **Jay Joseph sees the turn:** Joseph, Jay (2006). *The Missing Gene: Psychiatry, Heredity, and the Fruitless Search for Genes.* New York: Algora, p 239.

230 **Joseph has compared:** Joseph 242.

231 **For psychologist Sharna Olfman:** Olfman, Sharna (January 25, 2016). "The Genetics of Schizophrenia: A Left Brain Theory About a Right Brain Deficit in a Left Brain World." *Mad in America.* https://www.madinamerica.com/2016/01/the-genetics-of-schizophrenia-a-left-brain-theory-about-a-right-brain-deficit-in-a-left-brain-world/. Retrieved on October 3, 2022.

231 **The recent return of the notion:** Saini, Angela (2019). *Superior: The Return of Race Science.* Boston: Beacon.

231 **In a piece titled:** Aftab, Awais (May 25, 2020). "The Degenerative Agenda of Explaining Away Genetic Research in Schizophrenia." *A Myth in Creation* (blog). https://awaisaftab.blogspot.com/2020/03/the-degenerative-agenda-of-explaining.html. Retrieved on October 3, 2022.

231 **whose Danish-American studies:** Joseph, Jay (January 18, 2016). "Schizophrenia and Genetics: A Closer Look at the Evidence." *Mad in America.* https://www.madinamerica.com/2016/01/schizophrenia-and-genetics-a-closer-look-at-the-evidence/. Retrieved on October 3, 2022.

232 **In his 1991 book:** Breggin, Peter (1991). *Toxic Psychiatry: Why Therapy, Empathy and Love Must Replace the Drugs, Electroshock, and Biochemical Theories of the "New Psychiatry."* New York: St. Martin's, p 106.

232 **In his 2003 book:** Bentall, Richard (2003). *Madness Explained: Psychosis and Human Nature.* New York: Penguin, p 80.

233 **Rosenthal admitted:** Rosenthal, David (1971). "A Program of Research on Heredity in Schizophrenia." *Behavioral Science* 16, p 194.

233 **Many psychiatrists now understand:** Ophir, Orna (July 28, 2022). "The End of Schizophrenia." *Slate.* https://slate.com/technology/2022/07/schizophrenia-diagnosis-history-dsm.html. Retrieved on October 3, 2022.

233 **recognizing that hallucinations:** Rosenthal, David, and Olive Quinn (1977). "Quadruplet Hallucinations: Phenotypic Variations of a Schizophrenic Genotype." *Archives of General Psychiatry* 34.8, pp 817–27.

233 **"grossly oversold":** Breggin 107; see also Joseph, Jay (March 2000). "Inaccuracy and Bias in Textbooks Reporting Psychiatric Research: The Case of the Schizophrenia Adoption Studies." *Politics and the Life Sciences* 19.1, pp 89–99.

233 **Breggin warns of "America-hating" globalists:** Breggin, Peter R., and Ginger Ross Breggin (2021). *COVID-19 and the Global Predators: We Are the Prey.* Ithaca: Lake Edge, pp 453, 719. E-book.

233 **decries as "child abuse":** Breggin, Peter R. (October 25, 2011). "The Diagnosing and Drugging of 'ADHD' Children—An American Tragedy Worsens." *Huff Post.* https://www.huffpost.com/entry/children-and-adhd_b_1026477. Retrieved on October 3, 2022.

236 **The brainchild of Robert Felix:** Smith, Matthew (June 7, 2016). "A Fine Balance: Individualism, Society and the Prevention of Mental Illness in the United States, 1945–1968." *Palgrave Communications* 2, pp 1–11.

236 **NIMH administrator Matthew Dumont captured:** Torrey, E. Fuller (2013). *American Psychosis: How the Federal Government Destroyed the Mental Illness Treatment System.* Oxford, UK: Oxford University Press, pp 67, 177.

236 **their outcomes considerably worse:** Barry, Ellen (February 22, 2022). "The 'Nation's Psychiatrist' Takes Stock, with Frustration." *New York Times.* https://www.nytimes.com/2022/02/22/us/thomas-insel-book.html. Retrieved October 3, 2022.

236 **Freudian doctrine of neutrality persists:** Zeavin, Hannah (Spring 2022). "Unfree Associations: Parasitic Whiteness On and Off the Couch." *n+1* 42. https://www.nplusonemag.com/issue-42/essays/unfree-associations/. Retrieved October 3, 2022.

237 **During his last year:** Barry.

237 **"health is more about":** Insel, Thomas (2022). *Healing: Our Path from Mental Illness to Mental Health.* New York: Penguin, p 221.

237 **"languish on our streets":** Barry.

237 **"Kennedy's call to action":** Insel xviii.

237 **the federal government has taken:** Insel 195–96.

238 **Some psychoanalysts are also coming to grips:** Zeavin.

238 **in the words of scholar George Lipsitz:** Lipsitz, George (September 1995). "The Possessive Investment in Whiteness: Racialized Social Democracy and the 'White' Problem in American Studies." *American Quarterly* 47.3, p 369.

239 **But there was one conference:** Zeavin.

239 **Beyond psychoanalytic circles:** Interview with Laura Anderson. January 24, 2022.

240 **A *New York Times* headline conveyed:** Bennett, Jessica (February 4, 2022). "If Everything Is 'Trauma,' Is Anything?" *New York Times.* https://www.nytimes.com/2022/02/04/opinion/caleb-love-bombing-gaslighting-trauma.html. Retrieved October 3, 2022.

240 **And as Aftab noted:** Awais Aftab, @AwaisAftab (April 21, 2022). ["One could say that it is only by defining 'trauma' so broadly and loosely that you are able to see it everywhere."] Twitter. https://twitter.com/awaisaftab/status/1517091153744650241?s=20&t=nM9mu2MWrwwmd9xXoMtNhQ.

241 **global Hearing Voices movement:** "About Us." Hearing Voices USA. http://www.hearingvoicesusa.org/about-us. Retrieved October 3, 2022.

241 **not always more effective:** WrenAves (July 12, 2022). "'Trauma-Informed Care' Left Me More Traumatised Than Ever." *Psychiatry Is Driving Me Mad* (blog). https://www.psychiatryisdrivingmemad.co.uk/post/trauma-informed-care-left-me-more-traumatised-than-ever. Retrieved October 3, 2022.

CHAPTER SEVENTEEN

247 **Mirsky et al. published:** Mirksy, Allan F., et al. (2013). "The Genain Quadruplets: A 55-Year Follow-Up of Two of Four Monozygous Sisters with Schizophrenia." *Schizophrenia Research* 148, pp 186–87.

247 **"We really were like little tin soldiers":** Cotton, Sarah Morlok (2015). *The Morlok Quadruplets: The Alphabet Sisters.* Scotts Valley, CA: CreateSpace, p 140.

247 **"just plain possessive":** Cotton 142.

247 **"As we grew older":** Cotton 141.

About the Author

Audrey Clare Farley is the author of *The Unfit Heiress: The Tragic Life and Scandalous Sterilization of Ann Cooper Hewitt*. She earned a PhD in English literature from the University of Maryland, College Park, and now teaches history and creative writing. Her essays have appeared in the *Atlantic*, *New Republic*, *Washington Post*, and many other outlets. She lives in Hanover, Pennsylvania.